The Paradox of Progress

James Willis MBBS MRCGP DCH

With a Foreword by
James McCormick

Radcliffe Medical Press
Oxford and New York

Radcliffe Medical Press Ltd
18 Marcham Road, Abingdon, Oxon OX14 1AA, UK

Radcliffe Medical Press, Inc
141 Fifth Avenue, New York, NY 10010, USA

British Library Cataloguing in Publication Data

A cataloguing record for this book is available from the British Library.

ISBN 1 85775 063 2

Library of Congress Cataloging-in-Publication Data is available.

Phototypeset by Intype, London
Printed and bound in Great Britain by
Biddles Ltd, Guildford and King's Lynn.

Contents

Acknowledgements

My father, when discussing relativity or the meaning of words over the washing up, inside the chicken-house he was making, or under the car he had in pieces; showed me how to take the broad view. About writing he said, 'Have something important to say, then say it as simply and clearly as you can.' My mother, with her experience as a theatre sister, and her enduring warmth, energy and idealism, from my earliest memories taught me the true meaning of care.

Joe Talbot made A Level Biology seem easy. Rebecca West advised me to seek a career in medicine rather than journalism 'so that I would one day have something to write about'. Harry Levitt electrified me in my one hour's statutory undergraduate exposure to general practice – and subsequently arranged my elective so that he, Hugh Faulkner and David Morrell (then a young lecturer in Edinburgh) could show me what I wanted to do with my life. Sir John Nabarro, my first chief, and Tony Danby, my GP trainer, showed me the meaning of good doctoring. E V Kuenssberg, President of the RCGP, took me out for a meal when I had been critical of the college and told me to keep writing.

Christopher Everett was at this book's conception and has kept me going relentlessly ever since. Professor John Bain and Professor Philip Rhodes encouraged my first, shy steps, as did Richard Holmes, Sheila Goater and Graham Bridgestock. Chris Elliot-Binns, Patricia Tomlinson, Bruce Thomas and Iain Chalmers all read early drafts and gave generously of their experience; Iain in particular had a crucial influence. More recently Bruce Charlton, Professor David Morrell and Professor Nigel Stott contributed ideas, support and encouragement. During the past year Geoff Roberts, Peter Burrows, Rob Lorge, Michael Taylor, Ian Williamson, Sunil Bhanot, Don Grant, Jonathon Montgomery, Alan Pattinson and Professor James McCormick helped enormously with the *Paradox of Progress* theme.

Janice Mayhew, Judith Hepper, Tom Law, Martin Dell, Peter

Ashworth, Rod Eckles, John Duckworth, Andrew Doughty, Sheila Opie, my two daughters Becky and Caroline, and my brothers Peter and Andrew; also helped and encouraged. My partner Sheila Green, and our staff, especially Ann Yates and Thérèse Keogh, gave me a happy, stable platform at work. Gillian Nineham of Radcliffe Medical Press took on my book, and Camilla Behrens contributed her expertise as my editor.

To all of these people and to many, many others, I extend my heartfelt thanks; they share any success this book may have but are not of course responsible for its failings. Only one person will share that burden with me; my principal collaborator and personal life-support system, my wife, who has never wavered in her conviction that we have something important to say. Whether we have said it simply and clearly is for the reader to judge. This book is dedicated to her.

Foreword

James Willis has written a book that is both delightful and important. It is delightful because it is full of the very stuff of general practice, not the technical problems of diagnosis and therapy, but the human problems of people in distress. It also provides a moving portrait of a man who loves his work. This is because he satisfies one of the few important criteria of being a general practitioner, 'he likes the human race and likes its silly face'.

It is an important book because it is about those things which matter but are ignored increasingly. James Willis' central thesis is that preoccupation with technology and the 'measurable', seen as progress, has led to the relative neglect of those things, no less important, which cannot be measured. Who at the end of this century extols the virtues of wisdom and judgement? While *The Paradox of Progress* is set within the context of general medical practice, it is immediately accessible to those with no medical training.

As is appropriate for a generalist James Willis has drawn on a wide variety of sources and the book ends with a stimulating and catholic Further Reading section.

This is, in many respects, a serious book, but the touch is so light and so often illuminated by wit, that reading it is a joy and the journey is fun. I would wish it the wide readership it deserves.

Professor James McCormick
Ireland
1995

1

Understanding

The true story of a night call sets the scene and is used to show why GPs, like everyone else, must be educated for life and not merely trained.

'What can I do for you then?'
'Oh, I don't know *what's* the matter with me.'
'Give me a clue.'

My new trick

I've just fallen asleep when the telephone rings. Not so deeply asleep that it takes me an age to realize what the noise is, but enough to give me that sickening feeling of being dragged back to reality. I reach across and fumble for the receiver, craning to see the glowing figures of the clock on the far side of the pile of half-read books on the bedside table. Quarter to midnight. It feels like half-past two.

> 'I'm terribly sorry to trouble you but my husband has just got home and he's fallen up the stairs and seems to have broken his knee. I wondered if I should take him to casualty or somewhere . . .'

Almost all the tiny part of my brain which has woken up is concentrating on finding ways of staying in bed, not to mention going back to sleep. The whole of this meagre brain power now focuses on the patient's apparent willingness to go to casualty. An appropriate reply is necessary. Think, man, think.

> 'Well, yes, um . . .'
>
> 'He's lying on the landing in agony. He can't move the knee and it's ever such a peculiar shape.'
>
> 'I see . . .'

I do see, that's the funny thing about it. Already, in spite of my sleepiness, I've got quite a clear picture in my mind of the scene on the stairs, complete with a provisional diagnosis and a plan of what I ought to do about it.

> 'I see . . . It sounds as though he's dislocated his kneecap.'

I wonder momentarily whether I could talk her through reducing it herself, then immediately reject this as a silly idea. On the other hand, it is hard to justify a fifteen-mile ambulance journey and then hours of waiting in casualty. And then getting home again. I know perfectly well what I'm going to do.

> 'How are you going to get him into the car, if he's like that . . .'
>
> 'I don't know . . . There's the baby as well . . .'
>
> 'I see . . .'
>
> 'I'm terribly sorry to disturb you, doctor.'
>
> 'All right. It's OK. I'd better come and see him.'
>
> 'I'm terribly sor . . .'
>
> 'OK – I'll be along in a few minutes.'

I put my jersey and trousers on over my pyjamas, hunt for my socks, check the bleep is on, receive my wife's sympathy, step over the dog on the stairs, through the front door, open the garage door, feel for the car door keyhole in the dark, open the door, start the car. Gales of laughter from all around as some late night Radio Four comedian shouts the second half of what must have been a joke. Listen numbly to the puns as I drive through the familiar streets past people who don't seem as anxious as me to be in bed. I find the house with the light on and the right number. The laughter is snuffed abruptly as I switch off the engine and coast to a halt. Left hand grasps visiting bag, right hand swings open the door, I pivot on my feet and stumble into action, pyjama collar flying.

No need to ring the bell, a young woman in a négligé opens the door as I approach.

'I'm really terribly sorry to trouble you doctor.'

'Upstairs?'

'He works as a chef, you see. He's only just got home.'

I climb the stairs. The chef/husband is lying at the top of the stairs in an agonized heap. He appears to have nothing on except a blanket. His entire being seems focused on his left knee, which he is clutching with both hands as it lies flexed under him. I go straight to it and he reluctantly relinquishes his grip. Exactly like my mental picture – the great, hard lump stretching under the skin on the outside of the joint, with the peculiar dent on the front of the knee where the kneecap ought to have been.

Trying to appear more confident that I feel, I start doing what I have been rehearsing in my mind on the way – straightening the leg is the key. I grasp the knee with one hand and the ankle with the other. I fix my eyes on the patient's face. I tell him firmly to relax. To let the leg go loose. Not to worry if it hurts – which his face tells me it does. Monitoring his expression, I begin slowly to extend the knee. I feel the tension coming out of the patella tendon, and the kneecap slowly yielding to the pressure of my cupped hand as it begins to ride up on to the ridge of bone it will have to cross in order to return to its groove on the front of the knee.

Picture for a moment the dramatic scene. The silent, midnight struggle focused on the knee. The patient, the physician and the wife, variously attired and grouped in a powerful composition. Two, perhaps even three of the characters struggling to keep bridled an almighty scream.

But suddenly, instead of a scream . . . a 'pop'!

Like magic, the patella is back in its proper place and the knee is its normal shape.

I breathe out thankfully and sit back. The patient takes a little longer to realize what has happened. He gazes incredulously at his transformed limb and gradually the tension begins to leave his body. In turn, his wife, who is bent over us, senses the relaxation and begins to straighten up – her face showing the beginnings of a sobbing laugh of relief. The patient tries out his knee and finds that it will move. I encourage him to stand up. (He is wearing underpants after all.) I tell him to walk. He walks . . .

It is the sort of moment when, in an earlier age, cigarettes would have been distributed and everyone would have sat around in a state of mellow, post-ictal contemplation. However, being enlightened, I make do with sitting down on the edge of their bed and writing up the out-of-hours visiting slip. I apply a probably unnecessary but proper-looking crêpe bandage. I give advice on what to do if the knee dislocates again in future.

> 'Thank you so much, Doctor. Can't we get you something – a cup of coffee?'
>
> 'Very kind of you but no, thank you.'
>
> 'We're so sorry we had to trouble you.'
>
> 'Glad to be able to help.'

Back inside the car and the cocoon of relentless comedy from the radio. I have a five minute drive home. I lock the car. The dog doesn't seem to check my credentials as I climb over him on the stairs. Neither does my wife when I get into bed and snuggle up. I have a nice, satisfying feeling about that visit. I avoid thinking about whether there will be another call – I don't like superstition but this is far too important a matter to leave to chance. I have left my clothes draped over the bedside chair ready for instant dressing for the same reason. Putting them away neatly is, I find, an infallible method of making the telephone ring at one o'clock in the morning.

I use my new trick for getting back to sleep. I concentrate my mind on a phrase I like from the Pié Jesu in *Fauré's Requiem*. I exclude everything else ruthlessly. I sink into the music. I join in and become part of it. I am asleep.

My new trick seems to work rather well.

Understanding

When I do something really trivial in surgery I often joke with the patient that it has taken years of training to perfect it. I sometimes tell children that medical students have to sit for hours in classrooms learning to say 'Mmmm'. And there is a grain of truth in the joke. There are so many different conditions in medicine that you simply can't be trained to deal with each of them individually. But when you encounter each one it always seems that it would have been better if you *had* been specifically trained in dealing with it. General practitioners are constantly meeting new situations and what they do is to apply their broad knowledge and experience to the situation and more often than not they come up with an appropriate action.

As it happens, the incident in the true story I have just told you was the first and only time I have reduced a kneecap in nearly twenty years of medical practice. I've reduced fingers, toes, fractured wrists, and am a wizard at pulled elbows, but I've never done a kneecap. I'm not sure that I've even seen a dislocated kneecap before, or even a picture of one. By no stretch of the imagination could I be described as an expert in the field of reducing kneecaps. And yet the extraordinary thing is that I had a diagnosis and a provisional plan of action in my sleepy head within seconds of the telephone ringing.

I take no particular credit for this, it is just the way all of our minds work all the time. They create internal pictures so automatically that it just doesn't occur to us to think that there is anything clever about the process. But in this case I happen to know that I wasn't recognizing a picture I'd seen before, and I wasn't following a set of instructions I'd learned in my training – the two most obvious explanations. So what *was* I doing?

What my subconscious must have done was allow the various facts of the case to interact with the complex store of information and experience hidden away in my mind to produce that mysterious phenomenon which we call 'understanding'. In other words it produced a model of the situation in my mind which fitted the facts as I knew them. I then used that model – quite automatically – to work out a plan of action.

And this model was no ordinary model. From my knowledge of anatomy I could see the internal structures of the leg, complete with the displaced kneecap and the stretched tissues. I knew exactly what the ridge of bone and the empty groove down the front of the knee would be like and in a very real sense I could actually 'feel' them. Even as I was imagining these things and trying out the solution in my model, I was taking into account the distance from the hospital, the wife's anxiety, the pain, the baby, the possibility that I was wrong, the need to be available for another call in the middle of it all. All these things, and others no doubt that I have forgotten or was never consciously aware of, were included in my model of the situation. And all before I had put down the telephone.

The point of this little story is to show that no amount of training can prepare us for every eventuality in life and that what is needed is a broad education and a free environment in which to use our common sense – the extraordinary ability which we take for granted only because it is common to us all.

2

Our distorted view of the world

When a doctor compares his memories of patients'
problems with the 'reality' of his written records of the
same problems, he can glimpse the distortions normally
present in his perceptions of the world.

'If I don't come back in a week – you can assume that
I'm better.'
Young man with a relatively minor problem.

Mr Brown's same old problem

The next patient hesitates apologetically as he appears round the
door.

'It's me again with my same old problem, doctor.'

'Oh yes? . . . come and sit down, Mr Brown.'

If you think the skill of being a GP is making clever diagnoses
and saving countless lives you are wrong. That's a piece of cake
compared with remembering who people are and what is likely
to be wrong with them. If I had met this chap in the street I
wouldn't have had a clue what his name was. But here in my
surgery I have two secret weapons – my appointment list and
my pile of notes.

Mr Brown is due in next, here are his notes, and in comes a

face which fits – Bingo! – I greet him like an old friend. (Most of my patients are old friends, there are just rather a lot of them.)

Now what on earth may his 'same old problem' be? . . . I slide his record cards out of their envelope and go automatically to the date of the last entry – eight years ago.

I look up doubtfully.

'Your same old problem? . . .'

'My leg ulcer – it's bad again I'm afraid.'

Sure enough, eight years ago: 'Leg ulcer' – the same old problem – how could I possibly have forgotten!

Morning surgery

Let me try to explain:

When I get to the end of two-and-a-half or three hours of morning surgery I don't have any clear idea what I have been doing – I just feel fussed and more or less drained. If you were to say to me, 'Tell me what you have been doing this morning', I simply wouldn't know where to start.

I could pick out a few things to tell you but they wouldn't begin to give the whole picture – just self-contained parts of it. I could say, to take an example more or less at random, 'Mrs Grey was very depressed'. But it wouldn't convey what it was like to be with Mrs Grey when her nicely made-up and smiling face changed and she began to cry.

She had come into the surgery at about ten o'clock. I was running a few minutes late, about ten patients to go, probably about two waiting already. When Thérèse had brought in my tea she had warned me that there were seven visits in already and that four were in the villages – more calls than usual – the whole day would be a rush. Also I had promised to do something this morning about Mrs Violet who had been wandering all night and had left a towel to catch fire on the cooker. Antenatals at one-thirty but fortunately only three this week. Afternoon surgery starts at four. (I'm not making this up by the way, it all happened this morning.*)

---

* I originally wrote this section that same evening, December 31st, 1987.

As Mrs Grey comes in I am still thinking about the last patient. I look up and see her face, match it with the notes and remember who she is. She sits down and tells me that the pain in her chest is no better – the pain killers have made no difference. I read the last note:

- *Right para-sternal chest pain. Neck and shoulder pain. No root signs.*
- *Chest X-ray. Try Brufen.*

Now I am right back with Mrs Grey's case. The way this happens is rather like the beginning of those old ultra-wide-screen films that used to excite us in the 'fifties. I remember that the performance would begin with an introductory sequence in black and white on a normal sized screen. Then, suddenly, a resonant voice would announce from loudspeakers set all around the cinema, 'THIS IS CIN-ER-A-MA!' Suddenly you'd have the music and the colour. The curtains would sweep outwards and the screen would appear to stretch and stretch until it completely filled the field of vision from side to side. There would be a thrilling sensation of zooming right into the scene and becoming part of it.

Big screens seem to have gone out of fashion now, perhaps the equipment was too expensive to maintain. Anyway, the same sort of thing seems to happen when you identify the memory file of a patient and then zoom into it and become part of it. Every-thing else goes, the patients and the problems that were filling your mind a moment before are displaced, or left behind, almost as if they had ceased to exist. It is as though each patient has their individual box in the memory. Each box is firmly closed until you open it and go in.

> 'We've got the chest X-ray back, Mrs Grey, and it's completely normal.'

She doesn't seem to think this is good news.

> 'Well the pain is still there.'

The telephone rings. 'I'm very sorry, will you excuse me a moment . . .' It is a pharmacist in the high street to query a prescription; there has been a confusion over the strength of another patient's Thyroxin tablets. Thérèse brings in the notes. 'No, it's definitely 50 micrograms . . . No, I'm quite sure about that. Thank you for checking . . . Thank you, Happy New Year!'

As I look back to Mrs Grey my perception of her problems changes instantly and completely. While I have been talking on the telephone her face has crumpled and turned red. She is crying.

I wait, taking in the situation, sharing her distress, feeling guilty for the interruption, consoling myself that it might actually have given her the space and the excuse she needed to drop her façade.

> 'I just seem so tired and ill . . .'

I spend a lot of the next fifteen minutes listening. I absorb what she is saying and try to fit it into a pattern which provides me with a way of helping her. I try to avoid jumping to facile conclusions. There is no perfect solution – that's what makes it difficult.

Shall I say, 'You're depressed – take these tablets. They'll make you feel awful at first but you'll begin to feel better after a week or so. See me next week'? But she has had antidepressants before and she is sure this time it's different.

Should I certify her unfit to start work at the beginning of term? She really loves her teaching, the new school is such an improvement on the old one where she was really unhappy. It would be a blow to her credibility to miss work and might make it even more difficult for her to restart subsequently.

But on the other hand she and her husband sat down last night and considered completely re-thinking their lives.

> 'Yes, actually giving up for good. It seems such a shame to have the children at home for Christmas and just not have the energy to do anything with them.'

> 'Well, OK, what about that? What about giving up altogether?'

But then she would miss her work.

And so on . . . I have got the picture, as far as I can. I have done all the listening I think will be useful for the moment. My

picture is based on the archetype of the over-stressed, demoralized, conscientious, idealistic teacher who has, as so often happens, flopped badly during the holidays. Add to this elements of
failure to live up to what she expects of herself as a wife, house-
keeper and mother. Add to this a moderately severe clinical
depression, possibly post-viral (although she denies any recent
illness). Don't forget the chest pain. I think she probably came
to me hoping for a certificate for a few days off work to ease the
beginnings of term.

I put the options to her: two weeks off work and review, plus
or minus antidepressants, or soldier on and see if the stimulus of
work pulls her out of it once she is started. Nothing to lose if she
is thinking of giving up anyway. Come and see me again anyway
especially if the pain gets worse.

She decides to soldier on. I know she is still unhappy as she
leaves. I feel for her but I don't know what more I can do.

I make a record:

- Feeling very run-down still — contemplating not
being able to continue work. Has dropped out of
jogging, keep fit, drama. Sure she is tired rather
than depressed.

- Reassured about chest.

- Try to carry on as much as possible.

Deep in thought, I put her notes in the OUT compartment and
press the call button. I confirm that the end of my mug of tea is
cold while I wait for the footsteps and the knock.

'Come in . . .'

In comes little Flossie Puce.

'I've got a bad froat 'n all spots . . .'

Zoooom . . . I plunge into my mental file for Flossie Puce,
everything else is flooded out.

Mr Brown's distorted perception

So it goes on. Patient after patient. Twenty-four consultations that morning; something like six thousand a year. That's excluding telephone calls, trips up the corridor to patients being seen by the nurses in the treatment room, not to mention home visits. A great many people, particularly when each is as absorbing in his or her turn as Mrs Grey.

I often think that if I could remember them all at once I would go mad. But they must be all there in my mind somewhere, along with the many others who were patients in the past, complete with the complex and emotional sagas of their lives and, often, deaths. And then of course my mind contains all the other aspects of my life. Not least the nebulous ideas I am trying to crystallize into this book. An almost infinite richness.

This is the glory of life. But when nature ensures that we only see a tiny fragment of it all at one time, nature does indeed know best! Every memory stays tightly shut up in its box until wanted. But the result is that we fail utterly, and it is just as well that we do, to perceive the total extent of what is in our minds.

The fact that the focus of our attention – the Mrs Grey or the Flossie Puce – is really such a very tiny part of our total experience, whilst at the same time being so important, is a mystery which our minds can simply never grasp, however hard we try to make them do so.

So when Mr Brown assumes that I will instantly remember all about his 'same old problem' – his leg ulcer – he is only showing that his mind separates things into compartments just as mine does. Being a sensible chap he normally gives very little thought to doctors. So he keeps that box closed most of the time. But when he opens it, the few memories of me inside it are almost all related to his ulcer, and since he doesn't know much more about me than that, he assumes that his ulcer will be a dominant part of my life. And before we laugh at this too much, just remember that we are all doing this sort of thing all the time, and that there are special reasons why this is having profound consequences in the modern world.

Mr Brown is right that when he is with me his leg ulcer is the most important thing to both of us. But we are both wrong in forgetting the vast number of other things which are important as well. The fact is that there are simply too many 'other things' to fit into the mind at once. But not just more of them than we think, or even *far* more of them than we think, there are more of them than we believe possible. That is the vital point.

More than we believe possible!

We don't appreciate this fact because we have no means of counting or measuring the contents of our minds. We are not even sure that such a concept has any meaning. We are used to dealing with things we can prove and count. And when we make records on paper or store them in a computer we can measure their number and the space they take up. In that way we can be sure about the total size of the store. But we can't do that with the contents of our minds. It is beyond the scope of this book to go into a detailed discussion of the reasons why memories cannot be counted up or even defined as discrete entities. Nonetheless, I do want to point out a fascinating piece of circumstantial evidence which we can all verify from our personal experience. It is the way we continue to be surprised by coincidences.

However often coincidences occur we go on being surprised by them. And as Edward de Bono has pointed out, the fact that we are surprised by something is highly significant. It signifies that we are unable to explain it in terms of our existing understanding. And that means that provided we have made the surprising observation correctly, our existing understanding must be wrong.

So, even though we usually exclaim that a particular coincidence is 'incredible' we always try very hard to find the mistake in our observation. That is why we say; 'My eyes must be deceiving me', 'Something supernatural must be going on!', or again and again, 'Isn't it a small world!' Any explanation, in fact, to avoid the real one, which seems to be out of the question because it is a paradox. But if we accept that coincidences do happen, that the world isn't smaller than we think it is at all but quite the reverse, larger than we can imagine all at once, and if we discount the supernatural, then we have to accept that coincidences are merely one aspect of the way things are. We are left not having to explain the coincidence, but having to explain our surprise – which is much more interesting.

The real explanation of our persistent surprise at coincidences is that the experience of the world contained in our minds is larger than we believe possible. This fundamental distortion in the way our minds model the world, born of their incredibly powerful but essential ability to protect us from what would otherwise be an overwhelming weight of experience, is perhaps the central insight that has lead me to write this book. At every level, from the simplest personal experiences to mighty issues concerning the minds of international statesmen, this same distortion applies. And at every level we remain inherently incapable of comprehending its extent.

The mind compared with a record system

This is the reason, to take another apparently trivial example, why I never tell a patient to 'stay in bed until I call again'. However sure I am that I couldn't possibly forget because the patient and his or her problems are so dominant in my mind at that moment, I tell myself that I could. And that if I did forget the patient would remember it until his dying day.

> 'If I'd done what Dr Willis told me to, young man, I'd still be in bed, and that was twenty-five years ago.'

Cackle, cackle.

Anyway, that was what an old chap said to me once about another doctor, who had forgotten to call again, and he told the story with the ease of frequent repetition down the years. I have always dreaded making the same mistake myself.

Often there's a great deal more at stake than embarrassment. Even a single error must be prevented. One referral letter not written after surgery, one abnormal cervical smear report filed without action being taken could be disastrous. And it's all too easy for it to happen.

So the first principle you have to adopt is to finish off as much as possible before closing the notes and moving on to the next patient. This is merely a specific case of the general rule, 'do it now', which applies in so many areas of life. But many things can't be done 'now' – any more than a repeat visit to a sick patient can be done 'now'. I often need to wait for results, obtain further information or simply move on because of other pressures.

Many things are better and more efficiently done in batches anyway, dictating letters is an example.

For all such things that can't be done 'now' the technique is to arrange for something to stick out of the subconscious to remind you. You flag the notes in some way. Perhaps you insert an action-marker card long enough to stick out of the top. Or you stick, staple, paper-clip or rubber-band a label on to the outside. Any signal you can arrange that will make the notes stand out so that they don't disappear into the 'subconscious' of the filing shelves. Anything, in fact, that will act as an incongruity.

Notice here the relationship between the things that have been flagged as 'outstanding' and the great majority of things that were finished off at the time. The latter are now neatly filed away, tucked right inside their respective envelopes, and the envelopes themselves will soon be back in the obscurity of the filing shelves. The result is that at the end of the morning surgery the only things sticking out in the notes, and because of that, sticking out in the doctor's mind, are the flagged incongruities. They are really a tiny minority of the things dealt with in the morning but they are the only ones which are still there at conscious level.

The great mass of finished work now appears to be as invisible in the mind as it is in the Practice record system, but in fact there is a fundamental difference. The mind is still subconsciously aware of the whole of that background experience. This is why the mind feels an inner exhaustion after the experience of morning surgery while the Practice record system does not. The extraordinary thing our minds can do is to concentrate on the few things flagged for attention whilst simultaneously remaining subconsciously aware of the 'everything else' that is in there somewhere.

The best storage system in the world

Almost exactly the same considerations apply when you are picking articles out of newspapers and journals. Over and over again when you have read an article in the morning paper, or a journal, you put it aside thinking that it is so interesting that you will return it to and read it properly. And you never seem to learn that you almost never do. The article is inevitably usurped by layer upon layer of subsequent interests. 'The interesting article is dead; long live the interesting article.' Over and over again. You just never seem to learn.

I have tried to overcome this problem. Never to close a memory box containing something I want to remember without arranging an action marker of some kind. When I read an article to which I really want to refer I have tried sticking a semi-adhesive label on the page so that it sticks out at the top. It works beautifully. It warns me not to throw away the magazine, it says on the label what the article is about and it directs me straight to the correct page. Brilliant.

So why don't I do it?

It's just not possible. If I did it for any length of time at all, I'd have piles of flagged journals everywhere and no time to read them. Like those video-taped television programmes we all have gnawing away at our consciences until someone boldly records something else, newer and even more un-missable, on top.

In spite of all these discouraging experiences I go on trying this or that system for organizing all the incredibly large number of things I am interested in at the time. But the lesson that has gradually dawned on me over the years is that the size and complexity of our experience is so vast that it will eventually overwhelm any system. And the better we become at organizing ourselves and arranging clever ways of coping, the bigger the eventual problem becomes. All we are doing is putting off the evil day of reckoning when we will throw up our arms, say we can't cope and decide to do nothing at all.

This is where the specialist comes in – he (or she) is sure he has the answer. He thinks it is obvious that you must restrict the field of interest by specializing.

What a cop-out that is! Just another technical trick. If you don't include everything in your perception of life then you are not really dealing with life at all, but an artificial model of a tiny aspect of life. A far tinier aspect, what's more, than you will ever be able to understand, however hard you try. Specialization is certainly not the answer we are looking for.

A generalist has to be a realist, he has to cope with the world as it is. He has to tell himself that it doesn't matter how interesting the article he is reading seems to be; it is extremely unlikely that he will ever look at it again. And that the tidiest place to store its contents is in his head.

As a storage system the head is far from perfect. But the fact is that it is the nearest thing we have to a solution to the problem of gathering and making sense of our experiences of the whole of life.

Another surprising thing

To re-emphasize the point of this chapter, let me tell you what I noticed when I grew a beard. I had it for about a year before I got fed up with it and shaved it off.

I expected people to comment at first, and they certainly did.

Everybody had an opinion and it was sometimes quite difficult to drag them back to the subject that they had come to see me about. I got quite used to the double-take as people came in and it was a sort of instant pointer to the fact that it was our first contact since the great change in my appearance.

Gradually, as one by one the patients updated their mental pictures of my face (I suppose), this reaction became less common. But when it did occur it was an instantaneous signal that it was a long time since I had last seen them.

The thing that surprised me was the mismatch between my mental perception of the time since I had seen them and this novel indicator of 'reality'. For example, when a particular individual entered my room I might get that old, familiar, sinking, 'Oh my God . . . Not him again . . .' feeling.

At that moment such an individual might seem to be dominating my whole practice, my whole life. An overwhelming feeling that his problems would prove as intractable and frustrating as ever. This Jack-in-the-memory-box would come bursting out at me and leer hideously as it wobbled on its spring.

But then, in the same instant, the incongruous signal, 'You've grown a beard!' Meaning, without any doubt, that I actually hadn't seen (and therefore hadn't thought about) this person for nearly nine months – which in other contexts seemed half a lifetime away. Certainly somewhere near five thousand consultations away.

'I must be doing this sort of thing all the time, without realizing it,' I would think. 'We all must. It must be terribly important that we realize it . . .'

It *is* terribly important that we realize it. That we can only glimpse the whole that is 'in there somewhere' through the tiny window of our conscious attention and that, however much insight we think we have gained, the view through the window will always remain distorted. It is only contact with real life that enables us to maintain a sense of proportion and balance by constantly reminding us of the reality which is hidden by the selectivity of our perceptions.

3

The distorted view of the specialist

The scene shifts to the relationship between specialist medicine and general practice medicine and similar distortions of perception are found to apply. But in this case they are worsened by artificial certainty.

'You could be right, Doctor, you see more of it than I do.'
A patient, told he has 'flu.

The Super Specialist

I was going to say too much again, I knew the feeling.

I had been quite determined to stay quiet for once but I was shifting about on my seat like an excited schoolboy with my pulse thumping away in my head.

I put up my hand.

The Emperor turned to me and smiled.

And I began to tell him that I thought he might not be wearing any clothes.

It was a Saturday morning seminar on cancer at the postgraduate centre of our District General Hospital. The speaker was a gynaecological oncologist. 'Oncologist' means 'cancer specialist' and 'gynaecological oncologist' means a doctor who deals only with cancers of the female reproductive organs. This is a field so specialized that it doesn't even include the breast. So he was a kind of specialist amongst specialists; what we sometimes call a Super Specialist.

He was an Australian, passing through Britain on his way home after a tour of meetings in America. Speaking with confidence and authority he said how he disagreed strongly with the British policy on how often to perform cervical smears (the screening test to detect people who may, without treatment, be going to develop cancer of the cervix). His view was that all women who had ever been 'sexually active' should have cervical smears carried out every year, not every three years as in Britain, and that they should go on having them every year until they died – presumably, one supposed, of something other than cancer of the cervix.

It was when he had finished that I couldn't stop myself putting up my hand.

> 'What you are saying is that every GP in Britain should do a thousand gynaecological examinations a year. Just for cervical smears. That is twenty a week. Even at fifteen minute intervals that would take up one hour of every working day for every GP in the country – before they did anything else at all!'

> 'Yes, all my colleagues in my speciality agree that this is what is necessary.'

> 'Then you are wrong! It simply isn't going to happen! You specialists really must accept responsibility for thinking through the consequences of the recommendations that you make. If you say that cervical smears must be done annually then any doctor who does less than that will be automatically culpable!'

The audience was clearly embarrassed by this exchange. If the specialist in gynaecological cancer said yearly smears, then surely, yearly smears it must be. But at the same time I sensed that there was a sneaking, instinctive agreement with me – and that people found this conflict between their heads and their hearts disturbing.

The next question was on safer ground in some inaccessible region of gynaecological oncology research where the speaker was outstandingly knowledgeable. Everybody relaxed. He was back in his empire and all was right with the world.

One of the local gynaecologists present at the meeting, a less rarefied specialist, who had known me for years, surprised me by returning to my question after the Australian had resumed his seat. In a kindly sort or way he said that he sympathized with my view but that I should appreciate that I was wrong.

I seized this chance to clarify my position. I said how much I genuinely admired and respected specialists and how much I knew that we needed them. But at the same time, I said, they needed us. The generalist's viewpoint, which took a broad view and weighed up all requirements, needed to be better understood. General practitioners, like people in many other walks of life, were surrounded by enthusiasts with more and more bright ideas for things that they should be doing and they found it completely impossible to do them all.

The speaker, I continued, had made a logical error which illustrated the point. He had stated that in Australia doctors who aimed at one-yearly smears had found that they actually achieved an average interval of only three and a half years. His conclusion from this had been that any doctor who was unwise enough to aim at three-yearly smears would be bound to achieve something like a nine year interval.

> 'Not at all', I said. 'The poor result from the annual smear programme is exactly what should be expected from a regime which is perceived by the doctors, and by the patients, to be unrealistic. In other words, against common sense. A realistic plan is always more successful than an unrealistic one. In Britain we aim at three yearly smears and we are trying to get down to the job of making sure that we actually achieve that target – for everybody!'

I reminded him that an earlier speaker had actually ascribed the rather low incidence of cancer of the cervix in our part of Britain to the effectiveness of the GPs' three-yearly smear programme.

To his credit the distinguished Australian smiled at this and was big enough to tell a story against himself to show that he understood at least something of what I was saying. He said that he had once stood in for an evening on casualty duty and had ended up admitting far too many patients to the hospital because he thought they were all seriously ill. No doubt that 'bigness' was one reason for his distinction.

The exclusive approach of the specialist

Here we have just the same relationship between the focus of attention and the unseen 'everything else' in the last chapter. And the same distortions.

At times we all act as specialists, looking at the world from a narrow viewpoint. But when specialists use their microscopes to magnify tiny details it is often forgotten that microscopes also exclude the surroundings, the context, of the field of attention. While it is natural to admire the magnification, we often forget to notice the accompanying exclusion.

That is why the professional specialist, while he acknowledges that it is the generalist's role to fit everything together and manage the whole, fails to understand the size and the complexity of that whole. He never has to confront the whole as the generalist must. And the result is that when the conscientious generalist attempts to do everything 'properly' he finds that the sum adds up to more than a hundred per cent and the pot of life overflows.

In medicine, individual specialists may think that GPs don't adhere to their particular enthusiasms because of laziness, or incompetence, or bad organization, or shortage of money, or ignorance, or something. What they never realize is that they can *only* be implemented in isolation. It is quite impossible to put them together with all the recommendations from all the *other* specialists to make a world which works.

Generalists often react to the advice or the instructions or the criticisms of specialists with exasperation, 'He must think that we don't do anything else!'

The point is that the specialist really *does* think that we don't do anything else. Or at least, nothing else which is important.

The super-distorted perception of the expert

Technical experts – of the kind so necessary in the modern world, let there be no mistake about that – share the same distortions of perception that I have been discussing. But when they view the 'everything else' that exists outside their own speciality these distortions are far worse. For several reasons.

Reason 1 Exclusion

In describing how my mind works while I am seeing patients in surgery I have tried to show the discrepancy between the apparent importance of the particular 'memory box' I happen to be in at the moment and the hidden size of the 'everything else' which is in the background of my mind. While I am concentrating on the current patient is it quite impossible to retain a grasp of all the other boxes containing memories of all the other patients. But nonetheless there can be no doubt that those boxes are 'in there somewhere'.

But when a technical expert concentrates his attention on a single aspect of life, there is a fundamental difference. He doesn't have the unseen background containing everything else. Other things are 'not his field' and he simply doesn't know about them at all. Exclusion is inherent in his specialism. So, far more even than individuals underestimate the size and importance of the 'everything else' in their minds, experts underestimate the size and importance of the 'everything else' in life. They tend to think it doesn't matter that they don't know about the other fields. Those things can look after themselves. They are other people's problems.

Reason 2 Large numbers

I have a fantasy that sooner or later there will be a night on duty when all ten thousand patients ring me at once. But they won't. Although the number of calls on a particular night can vary between none and six, it virtually never goes higher than that. The rules of nature seem to prevent it. The number never reaches ten, for example; even once, just for the hell of it. Let alone a thousand. If you average the calls over a month or so the variation is even less, a factor of three at the most. And if you average the calls over a year the variation drops to a few per cent. And it really is very difficult to understand quite why.

In the same way, when people analyse the combined experience of many hundreds of doctors on duty, the number of patients who will ring on a particular night can be predicted with something approaching certainty.

But it is a remarkable fact that although the overall proportion (or likelihood) remains the same, whether or not a particular individual will ring on a particular night appears to be entirely random.

It is a feature of the modern world that decisions tend to be taken by remote experts and to be based on the near-certainties of the statistical analysis of large numbers. But front-line workers such as GPs operate amongst the random events of the individual scale. For example, although I can say almost exactly what proportion of smokers will suffer heart attacks in a given period, that doesn't help me at all in telling the smoker sitting in front of me whether he will be one of the ones affected.*

It is a commonplace in medicine that the non-smoker who suffers a massive heart attack doesn't feel the least bit better for the knowledge that his misfortune was very unlikely. He is rather like Jonathan Clay, the driver who, in the rhyme, 'died maintaining his right of way' and who, although he'd been 'right all along' was 'just as dead as if he'd been wrong'.

Reason 3 Retrospect

The most time-honoured method of lending events an illusion of certainty is to view them in retrospect. Since retrospect is nothing less than the difference between history and real life it is important to recognize the illusion. We base almost all our decisions about the future on our perceptions of the past and this matter is so important that I want to illustrate it in some detail.

Consider how very easy it is to define terminal illness in retrospect. When we look back on the last weeks of life of somebody who has died, we can say with total confidence that he or she was suffering, during that time, from a terminal illness.

You may think this is obvious, but believe me, it isn't.

It is easy to pronounce upon the special care and counselling,

---

* The parallel with the phenomenon of radioactive decay is irresistible. Although there is no way of saying whether a particular atom in a specimen of a radioactive isotope will decay now, in a week's time, or in a thousand million years' time; on the large scale there is an overall, measurable probability of these events occurring. Thus, it is possible to predict the half-life of the isotope (the time it will take for half the atoms to decay) with great precision.

for example, that a dead patient should have had during that terminal illness, in total confidence that he or she isn't going to sit up, wink at you and settle down to a few more years of life.

I once had a dear patient who had revealed her breast cancer to me when it was already at a very advanced stage. Almost straight away it was clear that the cancer had spread to bones all over her body and to her lungs. Within a few weeks her left arm broke below the shoulder through the weakened bone and when she came home again after having the arm repaired her right thigh bone did the same thing. When that had been repaired she became short of breath and I had to remove a litre of fluid from one of her lungs and more than half a litre from the other. She was such a tiny person that there had been very little more room for air.

If anybody ever appeared to be terminally ill, she did, and I told her so. She accepted this with the calmness and bravery which is the rule rather than the exception and which it is such a privilege to witness.

Her friends came from far and wide and her family came home from abroad to say goodbye to her. But she just went on. She had the most incredible and humbling faith. She said that with God's help, and Doctor Wilson, she would be all right. (The first time she said this I didn't want to spoil the moment by pointing out that she had got my name wrong, and when she continued to repeat it for months afterwards it just had to be God and Doctor Wilson who got the credit.) I visited her once a week, usually doing very little for her, always thinking it was near the end. Her family came back the next summer to say goodbye to her again but the illness seemed to go into suspended animation in a way which could never have been predicted from the treatment she was on. Almost a second whole year went by before she went into her final decline and died peacefully in our little GP ward half a mile from her home.

This is what life is really like. It holds infinite richness and variety as we live it but when we look back our minds select the things that actually happened and totally exclude the myriad things that might have happened but didn't. Again and again we forget that all those other possibilities existed at the time and it all seems so much simpler and so much more fixed than it really was.

I think this largely explains why front-line jobs such as general practice are so much more stressful than external observers understand. Moving forwards through life you continually confront a legion of open possibilities. But as each moment of choice or chance passes, the possibilities continually collapse down to leave behind the single narrow path that you have actually followed.

And once again we have just the same contrast of scale between the focus of attention and the 'everything else', the things that actually happened and the things that might have happened. And here again the 'everything else' is invisible, at least in retrospect. Life is a constant movement towards open possibilities which are closed for ever by the cutting edge of time.

Imagine one duty Sunday. It's lunch time and we are just starting dessert when the telephone rings . . .

> 'My Daddy has just collapsed, please come.'
>
> 'OK, I'll be with you straight away. What's the address?'
>
> 'Please come quickly, my Daddy is ill.'
>
> 'Yes, but where are you?'
>
> 'Please *hurry*, Mummy asked me to get you as quickly as possible.'
>
> 'Now look, I can't come until you tell me who you are and where I've got to come to . . .'

He tells me in the end. Through a mixture of luck and daring I negotiate the country lanes unscathed and arrive, tingling. The boy is at the gate and I follow him up the stairs at a run.

Daddy is lying on his face in the bathroom, looking distinctly dead. I kneel down over him. No pulse. Pupils dilated. Certainly dead. I try to look as if I'm doing something useful. I glance back over my shoulder and desperately search for words to begin to break the news to the poor wife who is standing anxiously behind me with her son – their son.

But she gets in first—

> 'I've got a homeopathic remedy here which is very good for collapse.'

There is a pause, and I begin to explain.

Just as I am getting back into the car my bleep goes off with the next call. So I have to go back and knock on the door, apologize, and ask to use the telephone . . .

Something like that can suddenly happen every moment I am on duty, and I know it. In retrospect I know that most moments they didn't happen. I know without the slightest doubt that they didn't. But although the memory is very much simplified in this way, the real experience of what it felt like at the time is in there somewhere, being taken into account subconsciously in my plans for the future. And when I view a coming weekend on duty with a feeling of deep apprehension, as GPs almost invariably do, I know something that an objective observer who looks at a bare account of the sort of problems I have dealt with during previous weekends on duty doesn't know, and doesn't realize that he doesn't know. The almost physical burden of things that might have happened but didn't.

The approaches to life which appear to hold the answers for the modern world are those which can be stated with precision and can be formally justified. One technique is that of the specialist who narrows down the world until some tiny aspect of it can be expressed in absolute terms. Another is that of the central planner who stands back from the unpredictability of events on the individual scale and views the world with the artificial certainty of large-scale norms and historical record.

It is difficult to say precisely what is wrong with these techniques. It is only through technical means that things can be measured and objectively evaluated. Technical means are in fact the very basis of rational argument. Therefore the technical approach to life carries with it an apparently unanswerable argument for its own validity. In more and more areas of life the superiority of the machine over the man appears to be self-evident; the head over the heart.

I'm not saying that artificial techniques don't have their uses, they do. We need them. What I am trying to show, against these formidable odds, is that the world also needs people.

4

The myth of the ideal world

All the problems of distorted perception that apply on the individual scale apply in a more malignant form when people are attempting to control the actions of others.

'When your blood pressure's normal, does that mean that your body's OK . . . You know, *throughout*?'
A patient who has just discovered she has a normal blood pressure.

The cyberman cometh

The Local Health Authority is just finishing off some alterations to the health centre where my colleagues and I rent accommodation. One of the many small jobs that still needs doing is the fixing of a leaflet rack on to a wall. So I am pleased when I notice one of the men fixing things on to the wall close to where the rack is to be placed. He has all the kit including an electric drill with a portable power pack. I stop what I am doing, go and fetch the leaflet rack, present it to him in a friendly sort of way and indicate the position of the two screws.

'I don't suppose you could stick this up as well could you, just over there?'

'Not today I can't. You'll have to put it through the office. I have to enter everything I do on this computer thing.'

In our health authority it isn't just workmen who carry 'computer things'. Community nurses and community midwives do as well.

In the past, one of the attractions of community work has been the independence and responsibility it gives to people. They don't have to work under the immediate control of superiors as they do in the tightly controlled hierarchy of a hospital. For a particular kind of nurse community work represents emancipation and they rise to the challenge and flower into wonderfully rich personalities who are a joy (and occasionally a pain) to work with.

It would be nice to think that community staff enjoy this freedom because those in authority realize its value. But it is clear that this is not the case. The new era of computer technology is demonstrating that this freedom and richness has not arisen by design, but by default. It is no wise insight that has recognized its ultimate necessity and value. It is simply that nobody has managed to find a way of extending the reach of central control out into the wilderness.

Until now.

Information technology is the answer to a central controller's prayer. In Britain its availability has coincided with two other factors; a tidal wave of management technology arriving, at last, from across the Atlantic, and unprecedented pressures to limit spending on health care. In this difficult climate it is entirely understandable that the central managers who have the job of co-ordinating health care have adopted the new techniques with enthusiasm. They genuinely believe that the quality of the service they see themselves providing is directly related to the precision with which they can direct the movements of their instruments – the workers. The result is here for us to see; the man with the drill in the health centre acting more like a robot than anybody would have believed possible even a decade ago.

At the same time we have highly trained and responsible nurses, who deal personally on a daily basis with life and death situations, spending hours of each week tapping codes into computers in order to describe their work so that it can be counted up and analysed and made more efficient by an Orwellian 'Big Sister' sitting at some unseen desk. I find this idea utterly repugnant, utterly naive, and utterly lacking in common sense. I think that both workers and controllers have become unwitting participants in nothing less than a madness afflicting the corporate mind of society.

I watch with increasing horror as the tide of this 'progress' begins to lap around my feet – as the Minister of Health begins to settle himself at the controls of his own new machine and gives a tentative tug at one or two of the strings with which he plans to bind me as well.

If we are to do something to stop this tide, feelings of horror and repugnance are not enough. If we want to improve the world we have to work within its rules and according to those rules feelings don't count. (For one thing they literally can't be counted.) So we have to provide a formal argument which will make it clear, even to the central controllers, that the world they are trying to create doesn't add up and that it never will; however long they go on trying to get their rules and controls perfect.

Before pursuing this task I will finish my story of the robot workman. He was apparently not 'programmed' to clear up the mess he had made. So he left brick-dust and debris all over the reception desk for our receptionists (who do not carry computers but whom we encourage to think) to clear up. The workman, of course, was himself a specialist and way above doing menial tasks. Such is the price of progress.

Stone checks

As proud new owners of our first car, a venerable Morris Minor 1000, my wife and I bought an owner's manual so that we could look after it properly. The manual was one of a series published by the *Sunday Times*. It was in its third edition, so it must have sold well. It was dated 1965. Here is what it advised us to do by way of routine, daily maintenance:

DAILY: Check oil level, radiator, petrol, tyres and lights.

Now, it wasn't at all clear what was meant by the word 'check'. Checking the oil level, radiator and petrol, we thought, was pretty straightforward. Messy, admittedly, but you knew what to do. But we never did find out exactly what to check the lights for. We guessed that you really had to make sure that they all worked but hoped that it would sometimes be OK just to check that none were missing.

The subject that kept me lying awake at night puzzling over was the daily tyre check. We had discovered from elsewhere in the manual that the enemy was embedded stones. And the problem, of course, was that at any particular time three quarters of the tread of the tyres was either resting on the ground or hidden inside the wheel arches.

So I would imagine myself rolling the car forward exactly a quarter of a wheel circumference, jumping out and rushing around with a penknife flicking out the pebbles. Then I would jump in again and repeat the process. Then I would repeat it again. And then I would repeat it again. Provided, of course, that I had left room to roll the car far enough forward.

To ease this preliminary to each day I tried to imagine more efficient methods, for example getting the car to roll forwards (slowly mind you) by itself, while I trotted alongside doing my checking and flicking, but they all seemed to have unhappy outcomes. It was a very worrying problem.

You can probably guess the admission I am about to make. It wasn't just that we didn't do this routine maintenance on our precious car every day. It was much worse than that. We didn't do it at all. And worse still, we got away with it!

Somehow (unless we just didn't notice) whatever it was that checking tyres for embedded stones was designed to prevent, didn't happen. I never did find out what it would have been if it had. But I still feel a little bit guilty about it. To this day I sometimes reach down and flick a stone out of the tread of a tyre as a sort of gesture to the car that I do, really, know how to look after it properly.

We still have that old manual as a souvenir, it is a good example of what happens when a specialist, in this case a motoring freak, gives advice to generalists (real people). Nobody in their right mind would think for a moment that the writer ever seriously intended his readers to carry out such daily checks. Much more likely he thought that it would be expected of him to give that sort of advice when writing a manual. That, after all, is what manuals are for.

To be charitable, he probably thought that he ought to say what he thought motorists *ought* to do – in an ideal world.

The ideal world

This is really a sort of game in which common sense has no hand. Everybody is supposed to agree about what they really ought to be doing but anybody who actually did it would be regarded as a lunatic. All that this kind of advice actually achieves is to worry frustrated obsessionals like myself with the idea that they really ought to go through these ludicrous rituals. (Frustrated obsessionals are defined as persons who would like to be obsessional but who can't keep up the necessary effort.)

So, when we say 'We really ought to . . . (do something)' we mean that in reality we ought to do it. In other words in the ideal world which is revealed by figures and facts we ought to do it. The point is that there is a hidden and unstated understanding that in the practical world we don't do anything of the kind.

The double standard of stone checks

Medicine, particularly general practice, is full of 'stone checks', many of them, as it happens, emanating from the organizations that provide us with professional insurance. And we GPs continue to pretend that we try to do them all because we have not got the courage to admit that the task is impossible. And we cannot admit that because we lack, both as individuals and as a society, a clear understanding of the selectivity of our perceptions. At the same time, however, there is an unspoken agreement that no doctor in his (or her) right mind would attempt to do all the endless things that are being urged upon them from all sides.

Just think, and be honest with yourself. How would you really react if somebody quietly and calmly showed you that he really could do all the things that you say to yourself that you really ought to do, and could fit them into a sane and satisfying life? Would you be pleased? Would you be inspired? Or would you find something to sneer at and make yourself feel better?

I remember a contributor to the training course for young GPs that I help to run. He was showing a video of himself giving trainees mock oral examinations – 'vivas'. In the video the first candidate was asked to list the medical journals he read and was duly castigated for not reading enough. The second candidate was quite different, he came out fluently with an extremely impressive list of well chosen journals which could hardly have been improved upon.

The put-down snapped back at once: 'Do you do anything else with your time?' Only the interviewer's back could be seen but the sneer was visible.

He was really only playing a game. He didn't really expect the trainee to read much at all – he just expected him to feel that he ought to.

The man who was magic

This reminds me of a short book by Paul Gallico that I once read called *The Man Who Was Magic*.

The story is about a medieval town in which everybody was a magician. Every man, woman and child in the population had some sort of trick or illusion which they could perform and they had an annual festival when they showed them all off to one another. Once upon a time a young stranger came to the festival. And the thing about the young stranger was that he could do *real* magic . . .

When everybody had performed their 'vanishing' acts and their handkerchief acts and their fire breathing acts, he took his turn and quietly unscrambled an egg. Slowly and undeniably, the scrambled egg changed into an unscrambled egg and then got back into its shell.

To find out what happened you really ought to read the book, it is beautifully written. Suffice it to say here that the people did not appreciate somebody really doing what they spent their entire lives pretending to do. They didn't appreciate it at all.

The unspoken agreement to pretend to do the impossible

There is a sort of tacit agreement in many areas of life, certainly in medicine, that everybody will pretend to do some things when to actually do them is completely impossible. In the past this unspoken understanding has served us well. But while our instinct warns us of the distortion of the specialist viewpoint our reason cannot tell us precisely why. The man who actually did all the checks in that old car manual would have been regarded as an imbecile. But for anybody to admit, even to himself that he wasn't going to attempt to do them would be an act of considerable courage.

We have a double standard here which is going to get worse as society gets more and more tightly organized unless we find a way of giving the corporate mind of society the equivalent of common sense. The hidden understanding (that it would be stupid to stick slavishly to all these special counsels of perfection) is based on common sense and it simply cannot be justified with the figures and facts that are increasingly being used to organize and quantify the world. Therefore it cannot be openly expressed.

In our brave, new, formally-organized world, all the things we say, tongue in cheek, that we really ought to do, are increasingly being laid down as things we *must* do, and people are being paid to make sure that we actually do them. More and more impractical edicts, each entirely justifiable from one particular specialist's viewpoint, are adding up to a society which is being smothered by the complexity of its own rules and regulations.

The Morris Minor manual with the advice about checking tyres for stones may have been written years ago but it would be the greatest mistake to think that we have since become any wiser. Quite the reverse. If we have finished wiping away the tears of laughter provoked by the silliness of an earlier generation of motorists, perhaps we can have a look at the 1993 regulations for the drivers of mini-buses at the tertiary college where I am a governor:

DAILY VEHICLE CHECK AND DRIVER REPORT

VEHICLE CHECK
These items should be checked prior to EVERY journey: Lights/ reflectors/rear markers. Wipers/washers/horn/mirrors. Oil/fuel/ water. Brakes, body, load security, tyres, wheel nuts, jack/tools, brake and electrical connections, number plates.

At one stage (the regulations may even still be in force, for all I know), all health personnel in our area were told to dress in gloves, apron, mask and goggles to take every blood sample from every patient. This was to protect from AIDS and there are all sorts of reasons, some of them obvious, why this is unnecessary (you don't catch HIV through intact skin), impracticable (time, expense, availability, etc, etc), counter-productive (people wearing gloves to take blood samples have been shown to prick themselves more often) and will worsen the existing problem of irrational panic in the community at large.

No matter; the primary object has been achieved which is to allow the rule-makers (who wouldn't dream of taking a blood sample, still less of driving a mini-bus) to rest easily in their beds. Nobody follows the rules that they dream up while they are there, but they can't be blamed for that.

The next stage in the madness is that if somebody somewhere actually does contract HIV from a patient – and it has been recorded occasionally – they may be denied benefits, support and sympathy because they manifestly did not follow the rules. Or somebody may have a crash in a mini-bus, and that occurs occasionally too, and get clobbered because it turns out that he (or she) didn't check the jack or the electrical connections on that occasion (and was honest enough to admit it). Nobody else did either, of course, but all the others got away with it.

Oscar Wilde put it well in *An Ideal Husband*:

> 'Everything is dangerous, my dear fellow. If it wasn't so, life wouldn't be worth living . . .'

So did a young motorcyclist patient of mine:

> 'Life is a very dangerous business, Doc, nobody gets out of it alive.'

Media scale super-distortion

Why do people who were presumably selected for their ability behave so stupidly – for there are countless other examples. A great deal of the explanation has to do with the sorts of distortion of perspective that we have been examining. In the case of the central control of contemporary society the distortions are enormously compounded by technology. Whereas individual people naturally base their judgements on perceptions of life on the personal scale, society as a whole tends to base its judgements on the unprecedented perceptions of what we might call the media scale. And while it might be thought that personal scale perceptions are quite sufficiently distorted by their selectivity, media scale perceptions are super-distorted by what we might call their super-selectivity.

In other words, rule-makers are responsible for large numbers of workers and they 'collect up' horror stories. Horrifying events, by their very nature, are widely reported and discussed and they make a wholly disproportionate impression. Because of the super-selective power of the media scale collective mind we think the events far more common than they really are. In fact the reverse is true and events are reported specifically because they are unusual. They become visible precisely because of their incongruity. The carnage on the roads, for example, makes relatively little impression whilst a single horrific murder galvanizes the attention of the entire nation.

So, judged by the realities of the personal scale, the likelihood of the events which are so preoccupying the minds of the controllers actually occurring seems so exceedingly remote that the complex, time consuming and expensive precautions which they have decreed to prevent them seem to lack not only proportion but sanity. And because of the selectivity of our minds, neither boss nor bossed can understand what is happening.

Rules are not solutions at all – they have become the problems

The cycle goes on and on. Once all the really common and important issues have been legislated for and solved they disappear from consciousness and we move on to the next level. Gradually, as the years pass and the world gets more and more buttoned-down the problems that the rules are being designed to prevent become progressively more remote and theoretical. Everybody gets the feeling that the world is grinding to a halt. Everybody, that is, except the tiny, highly selected groups of people who dictate each different category of rules . . .

The committees that are formed to create these ever more complex rules and regulations are themselves the product of a selective process of formidable hidden power. Their members are chosen specifically because they have the necessary specialized views of life. Even if a measure were to be proposed of such obvious imbecility that only half a dozen people in the world thought it would be a good idea, the committee, time and time again, will turn out to consist of those six people. This is partly because nobody else is prepared to waste their time with it but mainly because belief in it is the primary criterion for selection. Thus we get European directives on the straightness of bananas. God help us.

When mistakes are made which gain media scale attention, whoever is unfortunate enough to be deemed responsible will almost always be judged according to media scale perceptions.

To take an example, as fire regulations improve further, serious fires in modern buildings are becoming extremely rare events. Uncontrolled fires in sky-scrapers hardly ever happen except in horror films. But when such a fire does happen, and the officer in charge makes the mistake of thinking it is just the two hundredth false alarm of the year and sends someone up to the fourteenth floor to check, and, as happened in 1988 in Los Angeles, to their death, people are inclined to think the officer was incredibly stupid. Even though those same people would probably have done exactly the same thing in the circumstances – and would probably have called anybody who actually ran a full scale fire alert for all of the two hundred false alarms a silly old woman.

This is a very serious problem and the answer is not just better fire alarms. We are going to have to accept that there is a level of safety beyond which people cannot reasonably be expected to go and which can easily be exceeded when events are viewed on the media scale.

The same applies to people in any walk of life in which they deal on the daily, personal scale with matters which may occasionally result in a tragedy which will later be viewed, and judged, in retrospect and on the media scale.

Teachers taking parties of schoolchildren on adventure holidays, social workers responsible for 'at-risk' children and others in similar positions have come under enormous pressure in recent years with catastrophic consequences for their morale. We desperately need more understanding of this or people are simply not going to come forward to do these vital jobs.

Doctors have been in this game longer and have protected themselves better than most. But even so, times are changing. Some of the risks that doctors are now expected to take account of are so phenomenally remote that they can only be regarded as 'stone-checks'. But that does not prevent armchair critics from throwing the book at the occasional doctor whose misfortune (it can be called nothing else) has been highlighted by the super selectivity of the media scale.

In many fields of life and certainly in medicine we have now reached the point at which the very implementation of some of the new rules presents far more difficult problems than the original problems the rules were intended to solve.

All doctors in the EEC are now supposed to record the date of purchase, source and batch number of every pill and injection they administer. It doesn't matter how many other things they are trying to do as well, this is the only aspect of life that that particular committee was told to think about. Nobody will follow the rule, of course. They would be stupid to try. But in the unlikely event of their being found out they will be in the wrong. Absolutely, definitely, undeniably and above all, *measurably* wrong. And when that happens the court that judges them won't be interested in the 'everything else' that they were trying to do at the same time, either.

And what was the problem the EEC rule was trying to solve? You tell me. I think it was a theoretical problem to do with something called product liability. I don't get many patients with that.

So the rules are not solutions at all, they have become the problems. And although that may seem funny, it's no joke, we have to live with it.

Of course some mistakes are culpable and those responsible must answer for them. Of course standards must be kept up and improved where possible. But while some control of dangerous activities is essential in society we have to find a way of deciding at what level to pitch that control. And to do this we have to accept that there is no correct answer – no certainty that the chosen level is right. Perhaps it would be easier for us if it was otherwise, but it isn't. The level of control will always be a human judgement. The media scale gives an artificial perspective on the world which has distorted that judgement and detached it from the practicalities of real life.

The greater danger is that people will react to these unrealistic requirements for perfection by abandoning their common sense and working to rule. Working to rule and not to life is in fact the only way in which individuals can hope to achieve perfection in their lives. Then if something goes wrong they can't be blamed. They were only doing what they were told.

We are trying to turn the world into a machine

Specialization has been enormously successful as a tool for human progress at both the individual and the cultural levels. It has seemed to be a perfect solution to the two great impediments to our making sense of the world; complexity and uncertainty. But by its very success in solving these problems it has created an entirely new problem.

Incompatible ingredients have been mixed together and they won't make a cake. The ingredients are on the one hand isolated, specialized fragments of life and on the other a network of defined, precise rules intended to co-ordinate those fragments. The catalyst which has accelerated the exposure of this incompatibility is modern technology, especially information technology.

The world is being de-humanized. We are trying to turn it into a machine. It won't work that way and the evidence is all around us. Civilization seems to be running into the sand and we are looking more and more to technology to get us out of it.

But that way leads logically away from life – it leads to a logical conclusion to everything that makes life meaningful. If we want to move forward we must go another way. Towards living, human, ordinary things.

Then we must create a new synthesis which combines the best of both ways.

5

Weekend

A celebration of the reality of life

'You're a remarkable chap.'
'Everybody's remarkable if you look closely enough.'
Conversation with a (remarkable) patient.

I have said how stressful a GP's work can be. A problem shared is a problem halved indeed. I end up a day with ever so many half problems. A weekend on duty can be utterly exhausting.

But that is nothing compared with the problems of a weekend *off*!

One of the features of the modern age is greater freedom and self determination for individuals. In some ways modern life is like a weekend – and believe me, they are not all beer and skittles. Weekends for a generalist can be a nightmare and I mean it. With all these lovely things that I could be doing, and all those dull things that I should be doing and all those other things that people tell me I ought to be doing, *how on earth do I decide what to do*!

I have the greatest difficulty choosing what I want on a menu – choosing one thing means you can't have any of the others so I go round and round in circles. Some restaurants only offer one thing and I recommend them – they are very relaxing. Obviously they are run by sensible people who understand and they are bound to cook well. Patronize them. Unless of course you are allergic to everything except quails – in which case you have solved the problem in your own way. Unfortunately I like almost everything.

So, if life is like a meal in a restaurant with a very large menu, what are we going to do about it?

> 'Wisdom consists in doing the next thing you have to do. Doing it with your whole heart and finding delight in doing it.'*

When an animal is faced with a dilemma it can perform something which biologists call displacement activity – an apparently pointless ritual action such as preening.

Humans do exactly the same thing; faced with a dilemma, many people will walk to the mirror and comb their hair. Or they will start doing some other quite arbitrary activity whose real priority would be way down in any rational list. The fact is that there *is* no rational way of arranging all the possible courses of action in a busy life into order of priority. Everything is relative, what seems important in one context of thinking can come to seem trivial quite a short time later. The problem *has no rational solution*.

The day on which I settled down to start this chapter was an example. It was a Saturday. Here is a copy of the list of 'things-to-do' which I jotted down on a piece of paper. As you see I attempted a simple classification to help me decide priorities:

Book:
>   section on planning a weekend . . .
>   priorities

Easy but time consuming:
>   mow lawn
>   repair pictures for waiting room
>   haircut
>   buy shoes

Necessary but not productive:
>   run
>   sleep
>   eat

Relaxing and fun:
>   squash with X

* A saying of the thirteenth century German mystic, Master Echart, which I once heard quoted on BBC Radio *Thought for the Day*.

swim/sauna
read
sunbathe
help Y with his boat building
light bonfire

Chores:
write letter to Z

Then I wrote 'Allocate time' and underlined it heavily . . .

That morning, as always, when setting off on my run I had unlocked the back door and as always, I had been irritated by the door lock.

For years it had been getting stiffer and stiffer and I was finding it more and more difficult to hold the key in the way that, with luck, succeeded in unlocking it. The catch itself was also faulty. When you turned the handle it withdrew all right, but it wouldn't spring back unless you rattled the handle and the door in a certain way – the door stayed shut because of the pressure of the draught excluder strip, but not very firmly. All this I did more or less automatically, but with subconscious awareness of an irritant – an incongruity, I suppose, in my world.

Replacing the lock was one of my lower-order priorities; things which needed doing but the time never seemed quite right because they had been that way for so long. Anyway, I couldn't think how it could be done neatly because the lock was fifty or sixty years old and it would be impossible to obtain a matching one. What I did do from time to time was to attempt to lubricate it by squirting graphite powder into it through chinks in its casing. This was only slightly beneficial and I was unable to do the job properly because the lock was held together with rivets – or at least it appeared to be.

Anyway, this morning the lock became my displacement activity as I dithered about what to do with my precious day. It suddenly occurred to me that if I was going to throw the lock away I might as well have a go at drilling out the rivets and see if there was a way of replacing them after I had found out what was wrong and possibly put it right. After all, there was nothing to lose.

So I went and got a little screwdriver to take off the handle, and then I went and got a large screwdriver to remove the three big screws holding the lock onto the door. Then I looked at the back-plate of the lock and saw, to my surprise and satisfaction, three screw heads. Obviously the lock wasn't riveted together after all – in fact it was designed to be taken apart. Furthermore, one of the three screws was loose and was actually lying free in its hole.

Things were looking distinctly promising, provided that the reason the screw had come loose wasn't that its thread was stripped . . .

I carried the lock down the cellar steps to my work bench. Making space on the work bench is an art which I perform by placing my forearm along the front of the bench and pushing. Sometimes this results in things falling off the back of the bench and this I take as a signal for the unpopular business of tidying up.

Happily this complication did not arise on this occasion and I sat down, removed the three screws and cautiously prised the back off the lock. It came off, to my further gratification, without the air being filled with flying parts.

The entire lock mechanism lay exposed to my view, lying in a bed of dirt, rust and cobwebs. The pathetic inadequacy of my attempts to lubricate it from the outside embarrassingly obvious; all the bearing surfaces were dry and rusty. But more than that, as I looked I could see what was wrong with it. The whole mechanism was meant to be held in place by the three screws which secured the back. But because one of them had been undone and the back plate had lifted away, everything inside had been slopping about, in and out of alignment.

I could see how a cam on the handle spindle was supposed to press against a steel arm to withdraw the catch. On the other side of the same arm a spring was supposed to press to extend the catch again when the handle was released. But the arm had moved up on its pivot so that both the cam and the spring had slipped underneath it. The spring was deeply scored by the improper action of the cam over the years. It was amazing it had worked at all.

The problem with the lock had the same cause. The mechanism was a pleasure to look at. A beautiful assembly of shiny, flat, brass levers, each with its own spring. Each separated by a thin brass anti-picking shield. But because they too had been free to slop about on their common pivot they had not always been lining up with the profile of the key and you had had to fiddle it about until they did.

I gently released the springs and removed the assembly, carefully keeping the order of the levers unchanged. The rest of the lock mechanism lifted out in turn and I cleaned it all before beginning to replace it. I lubricated the bearing surfaces with a little grease and the lever mechanism with graphite powder, which is the best thing for locks because it isn't sticky and doesn't trap dirt. I pushed the catch arm right down on its pivot with the cam pressing on one side and the spring safely on the other.

When everything was in place and I had shown interested members of the family, I put the back on again and began to tighten the screws. To my delight the whole thing pulled up into perfect alignment as the screws went home. I made sure they were tight enough not to come undone again and then tried the key. Sure enough, it turned with the mellow smoothness of a good old wine – the solid clunk of a mechanism happy with itself. Not just good as new but better than new. Any roughness worn off by years of use.

Mounted back on the door, with one of the three big screws which had been loose replaced by a bigger one, with its brass handles polished brightly, the job was done; done to perfection. Complete. That 'box' was closed. And, as it happened, locked.

I felt a completely different person and I went up to the computer for the next three hours with a sense of inner peace out of all proportion to the real significance of what I had done.

It didn't matter in the least that the job hadn't even been on my list. Although I wrote the original of this section straight away after the event, that is now months ago and the smoothness of the lock mechanism is still giving me pleasure every day. Who can possibly say that it wasn't a good use of my time?

What I am trying to show here is how different the practice of real life is from the theory – how much more subtle, indefinable and irrational. And yet how much more valid.

It seems to me that as we move into a more and more rational and tightly organized world this validity, this humanity is being destroyed. If things go on as they are, it seems as though our lives will soon come stamped with a label which says *do not open – no user-serviceable parts inside*, and that we will have to live those lives in a sterile, defined, absolutely safe and utterly dull and unrewarding way. A modern lock isn't made so that you can open it and mend it, nobody has the time, you just throw it away and buy a new one. Then you can spend the time you saved 'enjoying yourself'. We call it progress.

This is why it is so important for us to think about the nature of ideas. Life is an idea in each of our minds. The reality on which the idea is based may be fixed and inanimate but the idea itself is incredibly complex and subtle. Life is vital and ever changing. It is too big to comprehend all at once. It cannot be pinned down and defined. To attempt to do so is to destroy it. But that is exactly what the modern collective mind of society is attempting to do.

Some such definition is of course necessary, that is not seriously disputed by anybody. The problems that we are addressing here are the widely sensed, but too little analysed dangers of too much definition. Let us continue to examine them within the particular field that I know about, the life of a GP.

Wasting my time?

What would you make of a patient who comes to me for reassurance a week before his regular six-monthly specialist review for malignant melanoma (the most serious form of skin cancer). He wants me to check to make sure the specialist won't find anything!

Is this a waste of my time, or an integral part of properly balanced care?

It only takes me a couple of minutes but gives enormous reassurance to the patient. The head says it's nonsense. The heart cries out that it is exactly what you would want if you were in that position yourself. Which is right? The patient's wife says, 'It's worth it for him to avoid a week of diarrhoea.' If it has that effect on her husband then surely it must be worthwhile?

I don't understand how or why my reassurance has this effect but I feel a sense of privilege to be able to give comfort in this way. I share his anxiety when he comes in; I share his relief when I find nothing. That may be part of the answer, I just don't know. I do know it happens – sometimes.

The principle which I try to go by is that each patient has come about a problem which is important to *them*.

Consultation involves getting into a patient's 'box' and sharing his or her anxiety.

At the time the stress and tension of the situation depend very much on that shared anxiety but an objective observer will inevitably judge the importance of the interview in retrospect according to the diagnostic label which was attached. In many cases the label may appear trivial because the things the patient was worried about were indefinable or easily ruled out. But that may actually have made the consultation *more* valuable in terms of promoting health and wellbeing than if I had discovered something dreadful.

A man recently came in white and drawn with anxiety. He had insisted on being seen in the morning because he couldn't wait until the evening surgery when there was more space. His problem was that he had found his xiphisternum – the prominent lower end of the breast bone which forms a hard lump in the pit of the stomach of most people. They are often very alarmed when they find it for the first time. When I gave this man the familiar explanation that the lump was entirely normal he practically capered around the room. He grabbed my hand and laughed and almost cried with relief.

> 'Oh, I'm so grateful – I was sure I'd got what my father died of . . .'

I remember another patient whose routine blood potassium estimation came back at 5.5 whereas the laboratory's normal range ran from 3.6 to 5.4. It had been unthinkingly declared 'abnormal' and he had been sent a note to come in for a check. When he came I was horrified to realize the significance that 'something wrong with the blood' had had for him. He had assembled his family for the weekend and they had indulged in a roast joint and a bottle of wine before he braced himself to come in to hear the worst.

This is what people are like

Like all my stories, these are as accurate as I can make them – this is what people are really like – it is not fiction. These stories happened, it is my interpretation that you may quarrel with if you wish. I think it is only through my human experience and values that I can understand these feelings at all. But I could never quantify and analyse them. I am certain that no central controller could evaluate them. I think the only real judge of their validity is the patient.

Several years ago I wrote myself a computer program to remind me to visit my elderly and disabled patients at various intervals. I have used it ever since because I give a very high priority to keeping in touch with my patients. But it is hard to think of any accounting system which would be able to measure the productivity of this activity which is so important to me. So either the accounting system or my priorities must be wrong. Of course in the quantitative, reductionist environment of ideas it appears self-evident that it is my priorities that are wrong and that is the view that a remote controller would be bound to take. But I don't think the customers do, and customers are always right.

Another patient – an elderly lady – told me that she was glad to see me when I called on one of these routine visits. She had been trying to pluck up courage to come and show me a breast lump. I had a look at it straight away and it was obviously a cancer. Not a very large one but that was what it was and I told her so. I said I'd put her straight on to some tablets which would shrink it down and refer her to a specialist.

The extraordinary thing was how pleased she seemed to be when I left.

> 'Now I shall be able to go out happy, now I've seen you, and I won't have to make up me mind to come and see you.'

The uncertainty must have been worse than the reality, even when the reality was the very thing she had been worried about!

As it turned out she was absolutely right, she responded so well to the Tamoxifen that the lump can hardly be felt several years later. And it certainly isn't that that is making her consider giving up her allotment to concentrate on her garden.

The practice nurses meeting

I am at a meeting of the thriving practice nurses group that had its beginnings in the treatment room of our Health Centre. Our six nurses have been the driving force from the start of the group.

My role as 'Doctor in charge of Treatment Room' has just been to shout encouragement from the sidelines and take a little reflected glory.

Tonight's speaker is a senior officer of the Royal College of Nursing and she has been talking about training. When she finishes one of the nurses in the audience tells the story of how she had suddenly found herself confronted by a man who had lost his entire family in a road accident. The burden of the speaker's response to this is that no nurse could cope with such a situation without a training in psychology.

I can't resist putting in my oar:

> 'What worries me is that saying that sort of thing will make people think that they shouldn't even try to help unless they have specialized training. Some people can do these things and some people can't, the main qualification they need is experience of life.'

She looks impatient with me and I go on.

> 'Don't you think it is possible that going on a course in psychology might actually make somebody worse at helping in this situation?'

She does not.

> 'Don't you think there must be some examples of training courses which are counterproductive?'

No, she does not. Training is training. By definition, it is a good thing. Like love or happiness.

I know many of the nurses agreed with me, they tell me afterwards. But they are just the workers, the boss knows better. Notice that if the original reply had been: 'You might have been helped by the education in psychology that I had'; I would have respected her opinion and agreed with her. What she said was very different: 'You shouldn't be attempting such a difficult thing without specialized training.' That is absolute rubbish. *Anybody* can give comfort and be a sympathetic listener – the more human and natural the better. Some highly trained people do it appallingly badly. Some do it very well, but even then it is impossible to prove that it is because of their training.

At least one of our nurses is, to my certain knowledge, a very effective counsellor indeed with no more and no less than her rich experience of personal and professional life to educate her natural ability. While I normally encourage all forms of post-graduate education I actively persuaded this lady not to seek further training in counselling when she raised the matter with me – though of course she would have had the final say if she had really wanted to. I thought it might well make her less effective and could hardly have made her better. I also thought it unlikely that those running the course would be ready to learn from her to anything like the extent that I would have been in their position.

Here again we have the crucial difference between *education* and *training*. Training is the sort of process you use to prepare a performing animal. It is an important instrument of central control. Education is neither of these things.

So that brings me back, more or less, to deciding what to do with my weekend, and to trying to decide what to choose from the huge menu in the restaurant of life. Our minds can sort these things out if we let them. They need education of course. They need to know about locks. They need to know about people. They need advice of all kinds. They even need a plan, so long as they don't take it too seriously. But however carefully we prepare our minds for life, like precious children, in the end we have to let them go if we are not to lose them.

6

Everything in life is relative

Almost nothing is absolute in life – but absolutes are
being used to attempt to describe our lives.

'Oh Tim's OK. There's nothing wrong with Tim!'
Young wife's response on being asked in passing about
her blind, diabetic husband.

'Did you win?'
'No – we were up against the Under Elevens.'
Captain of the Under Tens team.

In cowboy films people are 'absolutely good' or 'absolutely bad'.
This is a conventional simplification which is absolutely unlike
real life.

It is easier to watch a streetful of young men being killed by a
glint-eyed household hero if you have first been persuaded that
they are all baddies. Somehow the fact that they may also be
daddies doesn't seem to occur to the avid audience, but in real
life it would.

The closer you get to real life, the more complex and subtle it
seems; the further away, the simpler.

Almost nothing to do with people and life is absolute, nearly
everything is relative. Nature cannot, by definition, be 'perfect'
and most of the problems of real life have no 'correct' solution.
It is therefore hardly surprising, indeed it is inevitable, that nature
has equipped our minds with powerful mechanisms for making

judgements on the basis of things that are not absolute but relative. In recent years mankind has increasingly attempted to use machines to imitate and improve upon the workings of the human mind. One of the results of this has been to reveal, as never before, the size of the problems that the human mind solves with so little apparent effort. Here is an example.

The absolute limit

One of my personal projects in our health centre has been the construction of a general health screening questionnaire. The idea is that the patient has his height, weight and blood pressure measured and that he then sits by himself at a computer and answers a series of questions.

There were a number of novel features of this system (which is what made it fun to design) especially the fact that the report was addressed to the patient himself with the clear implication that it was his life and his choice about whether he followed the advice given. The point I want to discuss here is the difficulty of defining the advice that I was programing the computer to give.

Consider the section on drinking. There is no problem about getting the computer to ask for information on daily intake of pints of beer/cider, glasses of wine/sherry and singles of spirits. From this it is easy to work out the units of alcohol consumed in a week. (A unit of alcohol is defined as a glass of wine, a half pint of beer or a single of spirits.) Thus for each patient you get a nice clear figure expressing their alcohol consumption.

OK, what do you do next?

If you are absolutely opposed to all alcohol consumption there is no problem. In fact you only need to ask one question:

'Do you drink alcohol . . . Yes or No?'

If they say: 'No', give them a good mark. If they say: 'Yes', give them a roasting . . .

But I don't find it as easy as that. While I recognize alcoholism as one of the most destructive conditions that anybody can suffer from, and a common one at that, I also know that moderate drinking is very nearly universal, great fun and is almost certainly slightly advantageous to health. Where do we draw the line?

We are helped by the experts because for once they broadly agree. There is a reasonable consensus amongst them (at the moment) that the upper limit of acceptable drinking is twenty one units a week for a man and fourteen units a week for a woman. This gives us a starting point for our computerized advice. Twenty one units for a man will earn a stern but friendly rebuke: 'The upper limit recommended for a man is twenty one units per week, therefore you are drinking too much . . . Try to cut down.'

The chap who scores twenty units (by drinking, say, a glass of wine less per week) scrapes into the category below. He is told: 'Your drinking is in the upper part of the acceptable range; don't let it creep up', and he goes off to celebrate.

If somebody drinks twice the magic upper limit – forty two units or more – he gets a real telling off: 'You are drinking *Far Too Much* . . . Get help with your drinking.' Wow! Worth keeping to forty one units to escape that!

The real problem comes at the division between: 'You appear to have no problem with alcohol' and, 'Your drinking is in the upper part of the acceptable range . . . don't let it creep up.' Shall we set the division at half of the magic number, at two thirds, or where?

Well the answer is that there is no logical way of making such a distinction. It is a matter of balance, a matter of judgement. We do it all the time. But try to make a computer do it and you find out what a subtle business it is. Compared with the human mind, computers will always be clumsy and unsubtle, and no programing revolution that is remotely conceivable, even incorporating the wizardry of 'fuzzy logic', will enable them to approach our sophistication in making value judgements.

Finally, before getting too hung up on the mathematics of these distinctions, have another look at the figures they are based upon. To start with, the recommended drinking limits are picked more or less out of the air. There can be no scientific justification for claiming them to have a validity better than plus or minus fifty per cent, not least because they are changed from time to time. On the other side of the equation, the figures entered by the patients are themselves only the grossest of estimates, even when entered honestly. (Any sensible person ought to be very sure what is going to be done with figures about their drinking habits before entering them honestly into any computer.)

So here we have another example of the mystical power that we attach to figures simply because they are figures.

Just not the right way to measure the size of problems

For a period of ten years or so I had a patient who was terribly crippled by rheumatoid arthritis. Both legs had been amputated and she had gradually accumulated complications including a severe stroke. Her intelligence was as high as it had always been but her speech was gradually becoming more difficult to understand. She typed by holding a padded stick in both forearms.

She once asked me what on earth the point of her existence was and I replied that she was the person who made everybody else feel better by being relatively worse off than any of them. Which, in a sense, I believed to be true. (You'll never carry conviction when you say things like that if you don't believe them yourself.) Anyway, it amused her at the time and I think it kept her going for a little.

If a patient has been ill for a long time he or she will be grateful for any form of relief (although, naturally, sometimes indignant that it was not provided earlier). If the illness is only just beginning and although the doctor may know that he is saving the patient from suffering, and even from worrying about the possibility of that suffering, the patient is often not particularly grateful and is more preoccupied by the side-effects, real or imagined, of the treatment. This is why syringing ears (and restoring hearing at a stroke) is so much more satisfying than treating high blood pressure (and turning people who feel fit and well into patients requiring regular medication and supervision, who all too often feel ill).

Almost everything in life is relative. We all know that happiness has surprisingly little to do with physical health. Some of the most miserable people are perfectly well physically and appear to have everything that they could wish for. The various joys and cares that people have seem to bear no relationship to any measure of absolute importance. An old lady may lavish as much thought and care on her tiny garden as a Dowager on a vast estate. The loss of a dog can disturb one man as much as the loss of a battle disturbs another. I have seen more than one full-blown bereavement reaction to the loss of a budgerigar.

I dare say that the problems worrying the Minister of Health as he sits at his desk in the morning have about the same relative importance to him as my problems have to me as I sit at mine. One of us may be dealing with millions of people and the other individual people. In absolute terms it seems clear that to one of us the problems must be millions of times bigger than to the other. But our instincts tell us that that just isn't the right way of measuring the size of problems.

Absolute quantities do not constitute truth

Take physical fitness as another example. To appreciate fitness to the full you have to know what it is like to be really unfit. My advice to anybody who wants to keep up exercise over a long period of time is to spend a decade or so early in life at a rock-bottom level of unfitness, as I did, and then find out what you have been missing. That gets you out on the cold mornings! Appetite is the same of course. It is so relative that when you are full you find it hard to imagine hunger being even slightly unpleasant. And tiredness. If you spend much of your time feeling mentally tired there is nothing in the world like relaxing when physically exhausted.

All our perceptions are expressed in these kinds of relative terms. After spending a day travelling high up in a mini-bus, when we get back into our familiar car it seems very low. When we listen to a compact disc recording for the first time the clarity is almost overwhelming; a month later we hardly notice it. A child who has never known kindness will be amazed by a smile. And yet we persist in thinking that absolute quantities and measurements are what constitute truth.

The need for slippage

General practice is full of problems which have no absolute and correct answer. This is what makes it seem to be a woolly, vague and inherently less valid discipline than a restricted specialist field within which certainties can be seen to apply much more directly. But general practice is a much better model of life than is any medical speciality. Life is full of woolly uncertainty. By undermining our respect for, and confidence in, the mechanisms by which we cope with this uncertainty we are making it very difficult for people in the real world to live their lives.

That is why it is so important to make a coherent, logical defence of the generalist approach, in spite of the paradox that the generalist approach itself is ultimately illogical.

The modern understanding of life contains a fundamental inconsistency. On the official, media scale we treat life as though it is a machine, which can be analysed, defined and controlled precisely. And yet, our unspoken instincts tell us that life is nothing of the kind, it is infinitely subtle, flexible and relative.

Real people, operating on the personal scale are forced to live with life as it actually is. Thus individual working teachers, nurses, social workers, doctors or whatever, have no alternative but to accept that life is a series of messy compromises.

Society as a whole is now being confronted with that reality for the first time, because for the first time it has the machines and the systems which it thinks it can use to control life at the individual level. So the hidden cop-out is being revealed. The shabby posture of media scale society has been to rely on individuals for the slippage upon which life is utterly dependent. And yet, when instances of that slippage are exposed on the media stage, the individual is ruthlessly sacrificed.

By permitting slippage within the National Health Service, GPs act, in a sense, like the cut-throats whom the outwardly noble Macbeth secretly employed to do his dirty work for him. We follow our personal judgement, educated as it is, rather than the rules we are nominally meant to follow. Thus we provide the essential discontinuity on the logical road which, in an increasingly litigious world, would otherwise lead every patient with a headache to the brain scanner.

In order to do this we have to take a series of more or less carefully balanced risks, all expressed in relative terms. In other words we use common sense. But if society continues to denigrate this process and begins to expect perfection, as judged by the false perceptions of the media scale, then doctors are not going to allow themselves to be rewarded in the way that Macbeth rewarded his servants. We will eventually be forced to work to rule and not to life, in order to defend ourselves. And society will be the poorer. For however detailed the rules, any attempt to live by them is inevitably doomed to failure because the kinds of problems we deal with do not have logical solutions. And in any case, as I have already said, the complexity of the rules which would be created in the attempt would be self-defeating.

At the moment the move towards ever more central supervision throughout society is gathering pace as quickly as the necessary technology becomes available. But ironically, as a direct consequence, the need for slippage in society is becoming more and more apparent. After all, the more refined the method of counting you use, the more clearly it reveals inconsistencies. It is already quite obvious from a personal perspective that technology and rules are a poor substitute for common sense. The question remains how long it will be before this becomes obvious from the media scale perspective as well, and how far things will have deteriorated by then.

Generalists must lie

This brings me to the answer to a question which has troubled me for much of my life. A remark which a teacher once wrote on one of my history essays:

'He who generalizes . . . generally lies!'

I'm sure the remark was fully justified as it was applied to my essay but ever since I have been worried about its wider implications as a criticism of the entire generalist approach.

The answer, however, is this:

'Yes. Generalists must lie. Controlled lying, or slippage, is the only means we have of coping with the complexity and the uncertainty of life.'

The slippage which our minds permit, the subtle distortion of the literal reality of the world, is not a failing but a necessary strength.

7

Analogy

The power of analogy.

'It's like a compost heap in my chest that's gone wrong, Doctor. I'm sorry, but it's the only way to describe it.'

Double meaning

Machines that measure blood pressure (sphygmomanometers), like all other machines, sooner or later wear out.

I tend to hang on to my old instruments even when they are inconvenient to use, so long as they are still accurate. This is partly through affection for the familiar and partly through laziness. When a sphygmomanometer begins to wear out it leaks air when you pump it up and you have to keep pumping while you are taking a reading. My sphygmomanometer-before-last did this rather a lot towards the end of its life.

I remember an occasion when it was being particularly troublesome as I checked an old lady's blood pressure. Listening to the air hissing out of the cuff as I pumped it up around her wrinkled arm I gently broke the news:

'Oh dear, oh dear – this poor old thing has nearly had it.'

Same sentence, but two contexts and therefore two meanings. Fortunately the old lady saw the joke.

A lot of humour is based on double meanings, or punning. It seems to be the abrupt switch between two contexts which the same remark fits that does the trick. The better the remark fits both contexts, the more ludicrous the contrast between them, the more subtle the trigger that changes the understanding and causes the switch, the better the joke.

What does 'ROM' mean?

Easy! It means Right Otitis Media when I'm being a doctor and it means Read Only Memory when I'm being a computer buff.

OK. A more difficult one. What does 'PID' mean?

No problem. It means Prolapsed Intervertebral Disk when I'm dealing with a patient with back pain and Pelvic Inflammatory Disease when I'm dealing with a lady with certain other symptoms.

Post Coital Contraceptive and Parochial Church Council seem distinct enough. Yet the expression, 'Thank God for the PCC', is apt to retain a *frisson* of ambiguity.

Consider the sentence, 'With a bit of luck he'll pull through.' This is the sort of light-hearted remark that I make when someone thinks their precious child is about to die of athletes foot. But what if one day I get it wrong and find myself listening to the same sentence being solemnly intoned by a coroner? Or by a prosecuting counsel? Or read it in a Sunday newspaper? What would it sound like then? In fact this is a risk I happily live with, like the risk of driving my car, but the point is the same; everything we say is ambiguous outside its intended context. Everything in life is relative.

Words are far more ambiguous than we normally realize. I originally decided to illustrate this point by saying that the word 'duck' has a clear meaning but that we all recognize the ambiguity of a word like 'kind'. Then I looked up both words in my dictionary and found that it gives sixteen meanings for the word 'duck' and only fourteen for 'kind'!

When I scribble an address on a request form for a blood test it has to be transcribed on to a computer by a patient lady. (Not a lady patient you will immediately understand!) Now, this lady works at the laboratory fifteen miles away and she doesn't know the street names in our town, and she makes many mistakes.

But if I write the same address in the same (or even worse) handwriting for our community nursing colleagues, they have no difficulty going to the right house. How come?

Again, easy! The community nurses know the possibilities, they know the context and this vastly narrows down the possible interpretations of my scrawl (which was once described unkindly as the meanderings of a demented frog).

Communication

It is an interesting characteristic of intimate, human communication that we give the minimal clues to our meaning that we know a particular listener requires in order to understand us. This enables us to simultaneously exchange subliminal messages of sympathy. In this way exclusive 'in-groups' of all kinds; from elite corps of soldiers to subcultures like those formed by drug addicts, signal their brotherhood or sisterhood with a deliberately exclusive vocabulary.

By using obviously unnecessary clarity you can give an equally subtle but equally unmistakable message of exclusion. For example:

> 'GOOD . . . MORN . . . INGE. HOW . . . ARE . . . YOOOU?'

would be offensive unless spoken to someone who was very deaf, or very dim, or to a foreigner who spoke very poor English.

At a family breakfast, thanks to a confidently-shared context of ideas, any one of a huge variety of inarticulate grunts might be correctly interpreted as 'pass the toast'. And an elderly married couple who have shared a lifetime together can communicate the most intense emotions with hardly a word.

In each case the form of the communication is matched, with astonishing precision, to its intended audience – and this requires detailed knowledge of the likely context of ideas of that audience.

Whistling a symphony

Similar considerations apply when we communicate with ourselves, for we certainly use words and other techniques to clarify, record and remember our own ideas. So, when you whistle a tune you know well you can hear it in your mind complete with full orchestra, massed choir and the feeling of a huge hall filled with an excited audience. Your conception of the fragment of tune you are whistling may include the effects of the preceding build-up and the climax that would follow in a full performance. Although they are just a few poor notes in the wind to an objective observer, in your own mind you can hear – and feel – a symphony.

It is the particular memory patterns which are evoked by the tune that transform it. The notes are meaningless without the context of memories waiting to be drawn into prominence by the action of whistling. For a passer-by who doesn't share the context, the meaning which is so rich for you is completely missing.

So it doesn't matter how beautifully you whistle, how much you wave your arms about, tap your feet and adopt an expression of rapturous abandonment. If a listener doesn't share the environment of ideas in his mind which makes the tune meaningful he won't understand. You may passionately want to transfer the whole complex of sound and feeling in your head so that you can share your love of it. But if your listener's mind lacks the appropriate ideas you might as well be describing St Paul's cathedral to a monkey in the jungle.

Even in your own mind, it may only be when you are in a particular mood that the seed of the tune can take root and flower. Sometimes it will mean nothing to you as well; on another occasion it may move you to tears.

GPs are specialists in communication

The point here is that to communicate effectively, or indeed at all, we must be aware of the knowledge base of the person to whom we wish to communicate. This mutual understanding of the shared context of ideas is of the utmost importance to human relationships and communication, and to society in general. It is a matter of knowing the language, in the broadest sense of the term.

You may be wondering what qualifications I have for talking about these things and what relevance they have, anyway, to the theme of this book. The answer to the first question is not, for once, that I am a generalist and therefore interested in everything; it is that if we GPs are specialists in anything within the field of medicine, we are specialists in communication.

The answer to why this is relevant is that the shared context of ideas which is so essential for communication is the same, albeit hidden, background model of reality that we have been discussing.

Analogy

A charming and courteous gentleman of the old school, a remarkable amateur naturalist whose encyclopaedic knowledge of plant names was slowly and tragically deserting him, stood with me in his hall ten minutes after he had found his wife dead in their shower. In his threadbare tweed jacket he swayed a little against his stick as he contemplated the fact that he had drawn the longer of the two straws they had held together for so many years. Slightly the longer.

'The sun has gone in. I always called her my sunshine.'

What can I say?

When words fail, we use analogy. An analogy has to be a word or phrase of which we know we already share an understanding with the listener. Thus we all understand the enormously rich complex of ideas and feelings evoked by the word 'sunshine' and understand deeply the significance of this description when applied by a husband to his beloved wife. Putting the human force of this to one side if we can, without disrespect to its author, let's try to analyse what is happening in this amazing process.

When the poet says, 'My love . . . is like a red, red rose', he is taking two concepts that he knows the listener already has and inviting him to allow them to interact. The intention is that the listener will take whatever idea pattern may be evoked in his mind by the words 'my love' (presumably a girl the poet loves) and expose it to the pattern which is similarly evoked by the concept of a 'red, red rose'. The automatic functions of the brain will then ensure that the two patterns seek out any aspects which, in the present context, fit together.

Countless ways in which the two patterns do *not* fit having been excluded, the mental image evoked by the phrase 'my love' is subtly distorted to incorporate appropriate aspects of the 'rose' pattern such as scent, beauty, summer, fresh air, femininity, etc. Describing the rose as 'red, red . . .' conveys further qualities of depth and richness and perhaps evokes blood and the heart. The listener places this new pattern on provisional status and awaits the continued context which may either reinforce these aspects, or alter them.

Sure enough, the poet continues by enhancing the image of his love by exposing it to further patterns of ideas: 'melody . . . sweetly played . . . in tune . . .'

How could any listener fail to understand what makes the poet so enthusiastic about his love?

How much richer a means of communication this is than if he had said, 'My girlfriend is incredibly wonderful!'

But how *infinitely* richer than saying 'My girlfriend is more wonderful than 99.97% of the female population aged between sixteen and thirty four in Chipping Norton and surrounding parishes!'

But the last method is the one by which the increasingly reductionist, literal, mechanical, artificial world in which we live *has* to communicate its ideas.

Imagine one of the increasing number of self-confident new managers listening to this poem, learning about it, talking about it, until he gets the message. His eyes light up. He starts to smile. He says:

> '*I see*! He means that his love is like . . . like a very . . .
> an *incredibly* . . .'

He stops. The idea is there, but he can't define it. He can't pin it down. It is too large, too delicate, too subtle, to fit clearly into his consciousness all at once. He can't *begin* to communicate his idea. The danger is that he will retreat into his simple, secure, materialistic world and pretend that he never really had the deeper experience. He will say:

> 'I have it, I will construct a twenty-four point rating scale
> for all aspects of feminine beauty and desirability and
> then show you how the poet's love measures up.'

Yes he will. Believe me, he will! I know because I've tried it myself.

Take this book. It is an idea. A large, subtle, delicate, complicated idea. Far too large to fit into my consciousness in one bite-sized, definable lump. You may manage better than me, but not much. People ask me what I am writing about and I can't say – I mumble things about it being bigger than its parts. I say they wouldn't understand unless they read it.

The point is that this size, this complexity, this subtlety is a *strength* not a *weakness*. The whole current ethos of our society, that things should be pinned down, defined, recorded and understood is, in this vitally important way, *totally wrong*.

If we think our machines are near to human understanding then we are like primitive tribesmen who think that their wooden images are near to being men. If we think that we can reproduce the functions of the human mind with a machine-like system of rules and regulations, however complex, we are deluding ourselves utterly. We need to look elsewhere for solutions to the inherent problems of progress.

8

The ocean of congruity

An analogy for the way in which we only notice the incongruities in life. And the way everything else remains hidden from view.

Me, to an old lady hobbling into my surgery:

'What can I do for you?'
  Old Lady:
'Everything . . .'
  And as she leaves:
'I wish I could have helped you more.'
'That's all right, Doctor, you've done what you can.'

The sensitivity of our minds to incongruity is so inherent in our lives that we take it for granted and rarely think how clever it is. Consider the ease with which we detect a tiny grain of sand when we run our hand across the surface of a table, or the way we can distinguish a particular kind of vibration made by an underground train.

The power of this filtering process is a matter of common experience. We all share the mechanism which ignores everything that is congruent with the existing image of reality in our minds and selects for attention the odd thing that is incongruent. Some of my patients have houses backing onto a railway line. If you comment on the deafening noise of a train that has just passed you are surprised to find that they haven't noticed it. They say that are 'used' to it. Yet a tiny, barely audible, incongruent 'click' in another room will alert them to the fact that an electric iron has been left on.

As I have mentioned, my patients reacted instantly and almost without exception the first time they saw me with a beard. In just the same way it is extremely striking how quickly people notice that you are wearing a new tie or a new suit. The fact that people so often stop what they are doing to comment on such changes itself shows what a high priority the automatic mechanisms of the mind place on maintaining their internal model of reality.

So it is an inescapable fact, demonstrable by mundane, daily experience, that any new observation or idea is compared automatically with a subconscious, background frame of reference, and checked with it for congruity. Only a tiny proportion of new ideas which stand out because of their incongruity are brought to our conscious attention. Thus the overwhelming majority of everything that happens in our lives is invisible because it matches with the existing pattern.

It is the scale and sophistication of this background image, this frame of reference without which nothing has any meaning, that I am trying to describe. And the hidden power and importance of the subconscious mechanisms which maintain it in our minds. And the vital need to incorporate such mechanisms in society's understanding and planning of the world.

But that is an over-simplification. What I really want to do is transfer my whole mental image in a lump, without being restricted to sending a procession of clumsy words trudging through your mind. I need an analogy to describe the true wonder of the mechanism which makes analogy itself work.

The analogy I want to use is along the same lines as the familiar 'tip of the iceberg' but goes further. Forget about the huge bulk of the iceberg which is hidden in the ocean – that's peanuts – lets think about the ocean itself. Imagine an ocean made up of all the things in life which are unseen and unnoticed because of their congruity. All the things which have been excluded from attention by the selective mechanisms of the mind and of society. An ocean, in fact, of the 'everything else' we have been talking about throughout this book. The tiny fraction of life which reaches conscious attention now becomes the beach which is exposed on the edge of the ocean. That is the picture I want to convey.

Oceans in practice

There are countless oceans in life, and they overlap, but I want to stay within the context of medical practice.

In traditional practice, the doctor used to sit in his surgery waiting for patients to come to him with their problems: One patient – one problem – one solution – another life saved: 'Goodbye – Who's next?' Those patients who don't come don't register in the doctor's mind at all.

This is the analogy in its simplest form. The unseen patients are the ocean and those who present themselves are the ones who emerge on the beaches – the only ones the doctor sees.

The old style doctors had one exception to this rule, the chronic visiting list. This was a list of about twenty or thirty patients whom the doctor had got into the habit of visiting regularly, usually once a month. Some of these patients were very ill but this was by no means always the case, many of the visits were manifestly social. Other people who might have benefited from visits never got them unless they requested one for an acute illness.

Whatever modern doctors may think of this arbitrary arrangement there is no doubt how much the patients, and the communities they lived in, valued it. Or how important it was to the doctors themselves.

Twice I have taken over practices from retiring doctors and each time the *only* aspect of the organization they expected me to continue was the chronic visiting list. Each time, before they left, they took me around to introduce me to as many as possible of the chosen few. Virtually the only administrative advice either of these retiring doctors gave me was the style of diary to use to organize the visits and apart from selling me the odd instrument (odd was the word) that was it. I emphasize this point to show what a disproportionate effort was required for the active organization of this tiny part of the workload of a traditional practice. The enormously larger proportion of what the doctor did virtually organized itself.

It is curious that although chronic visiting lists are now unfashionable, other forms of active, doctor-initiated medical care are distinctly in vogue. The old, passive style of practice, in fact, tends to be referred to disparagingly as 'merely satisfying patients' demands'. The very term 'demands' is loaded with innuendo and 'satisfying' demands is seen to be a doubly spineless activity for a modern doctor. Especially when it is compared to the active organization of childhood immunizations and developmental checks, well-woman checks, well-man checks, old peoples' checks, cervical smear checks, blood pressure checks, breast checks, cholesterol checks. Every year somebody makes their name by checking something new. I plan to introduce alopecia* screening (with pre-emptive counselling) to a grateful world when time permits.

The new trend has been dignified with its own jargon. 'Proactive care', organized from the centre, is seen to be more important than 're-active care' which is diffuse and unmeasurable. Meanwhile politicians capitalize on the illusion that a health service can remove the need for a sickness service by somehow abolishing illness. Doesn't it all sound wonderful!

The new style of practice has many bonuses for the doctor. He feels he is in charge, he gets appreciation from the patients who feel that he is looking after them, he feels that his work is more purposeful, he can measure what he is doing. He can define his job and prove that he is doing it well! Not least, he has discovered that all these items can be identified and charged for. Cheques for checks indeed.

Doctors throughout the western world have learned the advantages of spending their time examining the healthy. Curiously, however, even the most sophisticated programmes of checks do not seem to have abolished, or even reduced, the need for treating the wealthy. The idea that preventive medicine will abolish illness and make everybody well remains what it has always been, an illusion. But it is an illusion which exerts extraordinary influence in the corridors of power at the present time.

* Baldness.

The enormous problems of active care

Of course there are advantages in properly organized preventive checks designed to serve the needs of patients, not those of doctors or politicians. But the snag that conscientious doctors are discovering about active care is that they have no alternative but to face the size of the task they are undertaking. They can't allow the practice to 'run itself'. It is no longer enough to be passive and allow each patient to come and open his own 'box' within the doctor's mind and then close it as he closes the surgery door. The motivation and the plan have to come from the doctor at the centre. And he finds to his surprise that the whole is far larger than he thought it was.

All sorts of difficult decisions have to be taken. For example, what to check and how often. Although we can agree, perhaps, that it is a good thing to have a full examination, there is no rational way of deciding its frequency. Once in a lifetime? Once a year? Once a week? And how full is 'full'?

Once doctors start taking the initiative in looking after their patients, they come face to face with these enormous problems. They sometimes long for the old days when the initiative came from the patient and there was no need for them to have any clear conception of the whole job.

The ocean of organization within a practice

Most modern doctors do take a succession of such difficult decisions and as time goes by the decisions accumulate into a complex system of organization for their practice. This complex system is another ocean.

But here the ocean isn't an unseen mass of patients but an unseen mass of organization – last year's exciting innovations which are now routine and which are no longer noticed. The incongruous parts of that organization which appear on the beaches of attention are exclusively the parts which have failed. And that, as we shall be examining in the next chapter, is pre-cisely what is needed for making progress.

Thus, when everything in the practice is sorted out and the loose ends of the patients' problems have all been tidied up, when the repeat visits and the follow-up of chronic diseases are organized so that they happen automatically, then the work seems to disappear from view. The doctor may actually feel he is under-employed. On the other hand, at times when every-thing is in chaos and he is overwhelmed with unsolved problems and chaotically bad organization he feels terribly busy. He *is* terribly busy – the beaches of his attention are crowded with writhing and incongruous bodies. But he is probably being far less effective than when he feels much less busy and his beaches are peaceful and deserted.

Although doctors ought to aim to be effective, not to aim to be busy, patients never seem to say:

> 'I'm so sorry to trouble you, Doctor, I know how effec-tive you are.'

Central control compounds the problem of active care

History has moved on one more stage in recent years. Central controllers have also seen the need for organized, active care. And for the very best of reasons they want to make sure that it is uniformly available to everybody, not just to those patients who have highly motivated doctors. (Central controllers, inciden-tally, are also unsure about whether they want doctors to be busy or effective.) So the controllers develop their own complicated ideas of organization. And that too is like an ocean.

The controllers gambol on the beaches of change, formulating their plans. But there is another important difference here. When they have handed down their instructions they turn their attention to the formulation of the next set of plans. The fatal catch is that they don't have to face the reality of implementing their plans and assessing the plans' effectiveness or shortcomings – they are above getting their hands dirty. They never have to hold the entire reality in their minds as a consistent whole. They don't think it is their job to do so. They are specialists. Their job is to selectively notice failings.

Put like this it seems obviously wrong, but it is happening all the time in the modern world.

Here, in microcosm, we have the whole story. The same problems can be seen in almost any walk of life, I have talked about the area I happen to know about. If we solve these problems we have solved the problem of co-ordinating individuals into a coherent, living society.

9

Making progress

We do not make progress by looking for final solutions, but by making successive improvements to the world, and to our image of the world.

'Mind you, you mustn't be *too* contented, progress comes from discontent.'
Elderly widower, in his tiny room, praising the National Health Service.

Everybody knows that a doctor makes a diagnosis by taking a careful history, examining the patient thoroughly, doing appropriate investigations and then reaching a conclusion. It is the time-honoured method taught to generations of medical students.

Strangely enough, what everybody knows is wrong – doctors don't work like that at all, or at least not very often. This is the sort of thing that really happens . . .

A shy old lady comes in and sits down – I haven't seen her for a while.

'I've got a little touch of . . .' She shakes her head and frowns: 'I can't remember what it's called . . .'

'Cystitis?'

She smiles with relief. 'Yes!' And then she looks startled. 'How did you know?'

'Just the way you said it.'

Patients would often be startled if they knew how accurately I can guess what they are about to complain of. But notice two things: First, I don't really know how I do it. I may think that I do and I may even be right. But I can never be sure that I'm right. What I am sure about is that it's a very subtle business indeed. Second, I didn't *tell* her she had cystitis, I *asked* her.

She might easily have said, 'No.' In which case I would have immediately switched to a new and better hypothesis and started testing that. Notice also that I had at that stage only discovered what she thought she had – I had to go on to find out what she meant by cystitis and then find out whether I agreed with her diagnosis.

We do exactly the same thing all the time in everyday life. Here is a very mundane example:

The doorbell rings . . . My heart sinks.

I am drying my hair having showered after a short morning run with the dog.

It is nearly 8.30 am and my wife has gone early to school. Becky's clarinet sounds from the lounge below. I am about to settle down to the second of the four whole undisturbed mornings that I have arranged for myself during this week's leave. My mind is trying to pull together the threads of the long-sought overall structure for this book. For once I know exactly where I am going to start. I am very conscious that I really ought to have got going an hour or more ago.

I think: 'Becky will answer the door – probably it will be the postman with something too big for the letterbox.'

And then I think of a more likely explanation – Mr T has arrived to continue painting the windows (he comes at this time to catch us before we go to work) – '*My* window!!'

My emotional reaction is instantaneous – a sick frustration in my stomach – in far less than a second from having heard the bell. Yesterday Mrs R wanted to clean the room around me, now how am I going to achieve anything if every time I look away from my screen and up to the hills for inspiration I find myself peering into wondering eyes two feet away through my window pane!

The clarinet stops – footsteps – silence – I put on my socks. I begin to relax. The silence does not fit with my Mr T hypothesis – Becky should have called me by now. Still silence. An alternative hypothesis gathers strength: Becky's friend Mandy has called before setting off for the college. But if Becky has for some reason chosen not to call me it would be rude to delay longer before going down.

The only way I can resolve the matter (apart from shouting) is to go down. I finish dressing and do so. On the stairs I hear the faint sound of a laugh from Becky. The type of laugh fits with the Mandy hypothesis. My relaxation is almost complete. I can see Becky's outline through the obscure glass of the inner door, but who she is talking to? I open the door.

> 'Hello Dr Willis, how are you?'

> 'I'm very well thank you, Mandy. I thought you might be a postman, a painter, a glazier or a plumber.'

> 'Well I'm sorry, I'm not.'

> 'That's perfectly all right.'

Continually jumping to conclusions

One of the contributions that academic general practice has made to medicine has been to point out that doctors work by this process of 'jumping to conclusions'. But not quite to conclusions; jumping to a series of provisional hypotheses is more like it, because the next and essential step is to test them. The process is rather grandly called intuitive-deductive reasoning but actually everybody does it all the time in situations they recognize. At first GPs thought it was something to be ashamed of but once it had been given a name it was recognized as a strength.

What I am pointing out is that these provisional conclusions are surprisingly accurate and provide an extremely efficient way of dealing with complex situations. It is another example of the pattern matching that our minds are so efficient at performing. Even in the most mundane moments of ordinary life, our minds latch on to a series of provisional explanations for the things that are happening around us. And even as they do so they continue adapting, strengthening, or replacing these explanations, from micro-second to micro-second. A process of utterly astonishing power and sophistication, when you come to think about it. Or when you try to imagine how you would set about imitating it with a machine!

In the past people assumed that the purpose of the human mind was to establish absolute truth and to guide mankind to Utopia. As a little experiment in thought, let us think what the design requirements would be of a mind whose primary task was quite different from this. A mind whose purpose was to hold the best possible image of reality and constantly improve that image in the light of experience. The building up of an ever more complex and beautiful image of the world, not the focusing down on narrower and narrower absolute truths.

Forgetting the practical details of how the thing would work, such a mind would have to be able to piece together and sustain throughout a lifetime a complex idea, or great hypothesis, to represent the reality out there which is being reported on by the senses. The crucial point is that this great hypothesis could never be perfect or complete, all that the design brief would require would be for it to be improved constantly.

The method by which we would be bound to proceed would be the same as that shown by Karl Popper to be the basis of all scientific enquiry. It would be by ensuring that the great hypothesis is tested constantly by exposing it to as much information as possible about the reality outside.

So first we would need some way of supporting, containing, holding the great hypothesis so that it was preserved and yet free to evolve (a gigantic challenge in itself, but not the present problem!). Next we would need as much and as varied information about the world as we can obtain. So we would want the best possible sense organs and they would need to be as mobile as possible so that they would report on the widest possible range of reality. That would mean not only arranging means for the sense organs to be transported far and wide (legs, bicycles, Concorde) but also building into the system an inherent motivation for that exploration to be carried out with energy and curiosity.

Next comes the really clever bit. The interface between the great hypothesis and the incoming messages about reality. What are the requirements here?

Simple in principle but unimaginably complex in practice. We want the messages to continually test the great hypothesis; to do this we want to find incongruities. In order to avoid being swamped by the enormous volume of data being collected by the senses, the mind will have to concentrate its energy on a tiny part of the data – the part which conflicts with its existing ideas.

It 'just doesn't want to know' about everything else. It wants to get straight on with examining and validating the discrepancies so that it can use them to update its great hypothesis. So, ideally, our design must make the testing process totally automatic and totally invisible.

So what we want is an inconceivably large, totally automatic, totally invisible testing process. That's all.

Oddly enough, our empirical study of the workings of our minds has already concluded that the thing they are most surprisingly good at doing is selecting for incongruity. And now we have an explanation of why this is so important – of why, in fact, our minds couldn't work in any other way. The great hypothesis is the same thing as the ocean of congruity – far too large to see all at once – and the incongruities are the beaches around that ocean. And the beaches, although relatively tiny, are the exclusive focus of our attention.

This concept of the way in which we improve our image of the world by constant small modifications is of the utmost importance. It has implications in every aspect of personal life and the life of a civilization. It applies equally well to the development of the ideas of society whether or not they are expanded to the media scale. It is important because it is so fundamentally different from the way in which we think ideas are developed.

In Chapter 4 I referred to an unfortunate trainee GP being grilled about his reading by a mock examiner. Remember the one who really did make a conscientious attempt to read the journals he thought he was expected to read? What is the next question the examiner asks (after 'Do you do anything else with your time?') when he has been told that the trainee reads half a dozen journals including the *British Medical Journal*? He says:

> 'OK, tell me something you read in the *BMJ* this week . . .'

The trainee's heart sinks and his mind goes blank. The examiner thinks he has proved that the trainee is either lying or doesn't know how to read properly.

What has actually happened is that the examiner has failed completely to understand how people index memories in their minds. He thinks proper reading produces something akin to a photographic record of the *BMJ* in the reader's mind which he should be able to read back on demand.

The reality is totally different and immeasurably cleverer than that . . .

Sure enough, people can teach themselves to memorize information in the exact form it was given to them. Some people do have so-called photographic memories. But this form of learning is far too rigid and far too time-and-energy-consuming to be a practical way of dealing with the experience of a full life (that may be why natural selection has not given us all photographic memories – they can't be a real advantage). What the sophisticated reader does is to scan through vast quantities of material allowing it to interact with his existing ideas. Everything which is congruous will be ignored, things which are new and incongruous will be selected for attention.

Often, incongruities are ignored anyway because they are simply too disruptive of basic ideas. We can't constantly be questioning everything. So attention to incongruities is itself selective, and individuals vary very much in their threshold of credulity. The system has been set up with a bias towards stability. This, as we shall see, is another feature of the human mind from which our society would do well to learn.

The mistake the examiner made was to assume that the new ideas which our trainee had selected for retention would be found indexed in the trainee's mind under the journal he had found them in. An elementary mistake, but the conventional wisdom. The ideas are actually neatly filed away, inside the most appropriate memory boxes containing the previously existing ideas that they had served to modify.

So if you say: 'What did you read in the *BMJ* this week?', the mind is blank. But if you hold a short conversation instead, it will constantly pop up memories of relevant things that have been read recently. Each time the reaction is, 'What a coincidence, I read something about that only yesterday!' (Notice that the trainee is just as surprised by the 'coincidence' as the examiner. The illusion is just as strong for him, that's why the problem persists.) Once again it is our old friend 'selection' at work. We underestimate enormously the extent of our reading because we store away facts in boxes in our minds as we learn them. We cannot open more than a few boxes at a time. But we have been taught to think that the literal, photographic kind of recall is the only kind which is really respectable.

The convergent, literal, photographic approach is a game with the dice loaded in favour of the examiner. It is a game invented and refereed by specialists and it only works in restricted fields of study. While it feeds the ego of the examiner it damages the should-be learner. It kills curiosity and is profoundly anti-educational. It is the most appalling introduction imaginable to a life-time of self-education in general knowledge.

I am certainly not saying that the mock viva was a bad pre-paration for the real examination. Quite the reverse. The pre-examination course from which the viva was taken as an example was extremely successful in its objective; getting people through their exams. The pass rate was close to 100%. But what the course was doing was to teach a technique of answering a par-ticular kind of question. What we really want to know is whether this kind of educational exercise makes people more or less likely to educate themselves twenty or thirty or forty years on in their careers. That is a question to which nobody knows the answer. All we can do is use our common sense, and there are no experts who can pretend they know better than the rest of us.

My common sense tells me that the doctor must not even try to memorize pages of information. The time for that type of learning was when he was at medical school long before and the basic skeleton of his future knowledge was being laid down. What the mature doctor needs to do (and in fact does do, whether he realizes it or not) is to constantly maintain and update his mind-image of medicine by exposing it to the whole range of experience and current ideas.

Fine-tuning a personal synthesis

The process is not that of photographing individual facts but the far more sophisticated and useful one of fine-tuning a personal synthesis. The fact that doctors, amongst others, do manage this process into the teeth of the head-wind of contemporary edu-cational effort suggests how very much better they would be able to do it if only contemporary education recognized this fact and exerted its undoubted energy on finding ways of enhancing rather than hindering it!

There are a great many implications once the reality of this model of the learning process is accepted. It provides an explanation for such diverse phenomena as perversity, negativism, criticism, the media emphasis on bad news, the restless search for novelty, and the emphasis on progress and change in human affairs.

It shows us why these things are necessary and inevitable and by enabling us to understand them, it may help us to contain them. And contain them we must in a world which is no longer a limitless jungle in which people fight ruthlessly for supremacy but a closed, finite community in which all must find a place and a purpose.

Critics

Although critics often anger people by being destructive and negative they are only doing their job. If it was their primary job to point out good things they would be called something like plaudits. But their job is to pick out incongruities and signal them on the media scale. Their name, rightly, describes their primary function which is to criticize and therefore promote improvement. They are one of many media scale equivalents of the mechanisms which search for incongruity in the human mind.

Critics are just one category of journalist. All journalists really have a common aim; picking out the areas of change and incongruity and highlighting them. A good journalist has a kind of genius for sensing the beginnings of a wave of incongruity building up on the surface of the ocean and then mounting that wave and riding it right up on to the beach so that he arrives just ahead of everybody else in a cloud of spray and glory.

It is just the same with fashion leaders and politicians. The game has all the exhilaration and risk of real surf-riding. It is a very delicate business to get right. Few manage it more than occasionally and even then there is a large element of luck. Don't forget that media scale super-selection operates to pick the winners and it is only in retrospect that their success appears to have been inevitable. Many promising waves peter out. Even when you are on a good one, if you move too far ahead and lose contact you are regarded not as a genius but as a crank.

An inherent need to question and challenge our ideas

So we have evolved with an inherent need to question and challenge our ideas. We restlessly search for better ways of doing things. In the past, civilizations which didn't have this quality of restlessness didn't evolve and died out.

But the emphasis on change has its debit side. We are easily bored by familiar routine. Motivation to do monotonous jobs, as we all know, has to be imposed by some kind of discipline, ideally by self-discipline. People will always be drawn away from the dull and the routine (the ocean – the important bit) by the lure of novelty. Those of us who are fortunate enough to live in the affluent world are selectively interested in the latest electronic gadget, the latest book, the latest clothing styles, etc.

New things, especially technical goods, may actually be inferior to the things they supersede, but that doesn't seem to matter. Nor does the fact that newness is so ephemeral. As soon as a thing is gained its precious quality of newness is lost. Then begins the longing for the next thing. 'To journey hopefully is better than to arrive.' 'When God seeks to punish us he answers our prayers.' We are like children. It is an embarrassing and unattractive characteristic which we all share to a greater or lesser extent.

MOLWA

Central controllers are every bit as subject to human frailty as the rest of us. But in the promotion of change for change's sake they leave us far behind. The problem is that central controllers make their mark on the world, gain prestige, importance and reputation not by preserving the status quo but by instituting change. I have long seen the need in Britain for a Ministry Of Leaving Well Alone (MOLWA).

This body would be the statutory equivalent of the automatic stabilizing mechanisms of the human mind that I referred to earlier in this chapter. It would have the responsibility for monitoring and appropriately rewarding people who have the wisdom to maintain successful and satisfactory institutions unchanged. It would allocate knighthoods for services to stability. It would prepare legislation to enforce durability of innovations so that any changes would have to remain in force for a minimum of, say, ten years except in the most exceptional circumstances. This would encourage a measure of serious thought before new ideas were introduced.

Another function of MOLWA would be to dismantle rules and regulations as fast or faster than new ones were created, with the object of limiting central control to an irreducible minimum. The place for innovation and diversity is at the local level. That is where we need the new ideas.

Whilst we await the establishment of this desirable ministry I would like to suggest the following tactic for teachers, nurses, social workers, or anybody else who is beset by professional changers. Just ask them, politely, 'What is the problem you are trying to solve?'

On the threshold of the ideal world

The remote controllers who would organize and change our lives and work rarely have any understanding of the subtlety, complexity and flexibility of the human decision-making process. They appear to think that the correct action in every possible situation can be defined in advance, and that it will be when they provide good enough rules. They feel themselves to be on the threshold of an ideal world when all these things will finally be sorted out, once and for all.

The corporate understanding of the remote controller is everything that individual understanding isn't. It is crude, inflexible and unchangeable. It concentrates on gross generalities rather than on subtle exceptions. It has a quality of blanket uniformity and yet is absurdly susceptible to the vagaries of fashion. And on top of all this it is applied with the ridiculous *certainty* which is the hallmark of the narrow-minded specialist.

People once thought that God designed men and women exactly as they are from scratch, and who can blame them? It was the obvious thing to think. We now know that God, or nature, or both actually proceeded by a very much better method – by the continuous fine-tuning and evolving of a great idea.

Since the dawn of civilization society has developed in the

same way, by the fine-tuning of an idea held collectively in the minds of men. Now, for the first time in history, we are trying to create a system of rules and technical procedures to hold the idea in a new and rigid form. We are trying to understand, measure and model everything using mathematical formulae and anything that can't be handled in this way we tend to dismiss as unimportant. The very attempt is bringing us up against the enormity of the task we have undertaken. We are gradually discovering that lists of things to do with life can never be complete, and that the thing which we want to know about at any particular moment is never on the list, because if it was on the list we would know about it already.

This may be a new discovery to us, but the ancient, hidden, automatic parts of our minds have been coping with the problem for countless generations.

10

Nature favours the generalist

Modern technology gives people a wonderful oppor-
tunity to develop their potential as generalists. It is also
essential to the modern world that they do so.

'Doctor's thinkin', Perc.'
Percy's wife, explaining a long silence.

Certainly not a back man

A patient once said to me 'I hear you are a back man . . .'

I hate being labelled, but if I were to choose a label for myself
it would certainly not be 'back man'. Presumably this patient
must have met somebody who had improved after I had manipulated his spine. Many GPs do simple manipulations in spite of
condemnations by real 'back men' who think that GPs can't
possibly do it properly.

People who do wide-ranging, general jobs are instinctively,
and without knowing quite why, unwilling to be judged by a
single criterion. The label 'back man' puts me in the same category as people who spend their whole professional lives doing
nothing but treating backs. I am then judged by that criterion
and (unless something is very strange indeed) found second rate.

But I don't feel second rate. I want to say – 'OK, I may not be the best there is in this field but I have a great deal of related knowledge and experience of the workings of the human body. I know my limitations and on balance, bearing in mind practical considerations of time and cost and convenience, my simple attempts are actually the best course of action for certain patients in certain circumstances. Particularly when the patients may have many other associated problems and I can't send them off to specialists for all of them without completely losing track of the patient as a whole person . . .' But I've lost you, haven't I? You still think I'm a second rate 'back man'!

GPs are caught in a crossfire of criticism in this particular field, which is why I have chosen it as an extreme example of the problem I am discussing. On one side we have the formidable ranks of the orthopaedic surgeons. These are the doctors who are responsible for the specialist care of patients with back pain.

For fairly obvious reasons orthopaedic surgeons see little of the common, minor back pain that GPs see almost every day and often several times a day. The orthopaedic surgeon's experience is restricted to a small minority of patients, selected because they have resisted simple rest, painkillers and physiotherapy, and often manipulation as well. So all the great unseen majority don't enter the specialist's consciousness at all. As a result the group of patients they see is far more likely to include people with the serious forms of back pain such as severe disc protrusions and tumours. (I don't dispute for a moment that this concentration is just what is needed to make scientific progress on treating serious conditions. I am referring to the distorted perception of experts when they extrapolate from their situation to that of generalists.)

The distortions do not end here. Nobody knows how manipulation works, there are lots of theories but the general consensus amongst orthopaedic surgeons is that none of them are valid. So, knowing of no mechanism by which manipulation can work they declare that it cannot work. They say, with the certainty of the expert, that the belief that manipulation does work is founded on illusion. And that those patients who believe themselves to have been helped by manipulation would have improved despite it.

Their attitudes are only confirmed when the occasional patient with a spine weakened by disease is made much worse by manipulation, even to the point of paralysis. Such cases are always admitted to hospital under the care of orthopaedic surgeons and feature in the medical literature. They are actually very rare indeed but media scale distortions apply and make them loom disproportionately large.

So there we have the orthopaedic surgeons. They think that any GP who manipulates spines is going through a pointless and dangerous ritual. Firing at us from the opposite flank we have the osteopaths and the chiropractors. Far from doubting the value of manipulation, they make their living by doing it all the time. Legions of patients, some of them doctors and some, I have little doubt, actually orthopaedic surgeons, testify to their effectiveness. But they have their own reason for saying that GP manipulation can't work. It is because GPs are not 'trained' to do it.

They have had years of specialized training, therefore they think they are the only people who should perform manipulations.

I continue doing occasional manipulations on certain patients, developing my ideas and my technique all the time, always a little uncertain that I am doing the right thing. I am unsure of the mechanism of my actions, but I do acknowledge my limitations fully. I have a life of experience of the ways of the human body and its pathological processes. And I have the trust of the patient. And when the patient, just occasionally, sits up with an incredulous expression and says: 'What have you done? What have you done Doctor, I can move again.' I sometimes smile to myself and say, in a competent sort of way: 'Just a bit of magic.'

But I wouldn't dream of calling myself a 'back man'.

Neither would a discerning three and a half year old called Gregory who pronounced the following recommendation just after I had removed a large splinter from his thumb:

> 'I'm vewy impu-wessed Doctor Willis, getting the spu-winta-woff.'

I'm quite sure he didn't want a back man, 'thank you vewy much'.

He wanted a 'generwalist'. And yes, he really was only three and a half. All my stories are true. He had picked up a turn of phrase from his father.

Definition

I had got to a late stage in the preparation of the ideas that make up this book without a clear definition of what I meant by the difference between a *specialist* and a *generalist*. In particular, I believed that the difference was a matter of degree and was in no sense absolute.

But I now know differently. Reading a book about the great British philosopher of science, Karl Popper, gave me the idea that I could define a generalist quite precisely, not in terms of what he does, but in terms of what he *doesn't* do. My definition is as follows. A generalist *never* says that something is of no interest to him.

Does that surprise you? Perhaps you don't believe me. But I can honestly say that I *never* say that something is 'Not my field'. There is a continuous spectrum of my ability and knowledge in different fields but at some level, I am prepared to be interested in *everything*.

My interest extends, for example, to Karl Popper work. And immensely worthwhile that interest has proved to be. It is a good case in point. Imagine we happened to be designing a curriculum for the training of GPs (and people are busily engaged in this particular aspect of progress as I write). If we ask, 'Shall we include Popper?', the answer might well be, 'No.' So then we would have to ask, 'OK, are we going to *exclude* Popper then?' And my answer would have to be, 'No. *Everything* is part of the training of a GP. And part of the job description of a GP, for that matter.'

So then you might reply, 'But we've got to do it. Defining curriculae and writing job descriptions are standard modern educational and management techniques!'

Quite so!

So, after all these years, I have found a way of defining what I mean when I say that I am a natural generalist and why, as a general medical practitioner, I set no bounds whatever to the ways in which I am prepared to help my patients. If an old lady needs help with understanding her central heating thermostat, if I am already in her house and I know how to help her, then I regard it as part of my job to do so. Many people do not. Some feel strongly that I should leave such advice to experts. I think that is nonsense.

However do we do it?

One of the things that I learned at school was that the more things I got involved in, the better I could do *each* of them. It has always puzzled me that this is not more widely acknowledged. I think people just think it is impossible because it seems so obvious that doing two things must be twice as difficult as doing one. They then simply reject the evidence of their own eyes that it is happening all the time.

They find excuses, they think that the reason some children are good at everything (I certainly wasn't one of them) is because they are simply brilliant. People just can't admit what they actually see happening, that being good at two things is frequently *easier* than being good at one. But if they do accept that this is what happens in real life the gate opens and you find you can move into a field full of excellent explanations as to *how* it happens.

I am going to give some of these explanations now. They are not particularly difficult or mysterious explanations, once you have accepted that there is something to explain. The first takes us back, briefly, to the beginning of the book, when we considered the relationship between the little bits of our memories that fill our conscious attention and the vast, hidden background of our entire experience.

Explanation 1 Bigger than we believe possible

It's not so much that the experience contained in our minds is large, remember. Or that it is *enormously* large. Both words certainly apply, but they don't tell half the story. The truth is that the capacity of our minds is larger than we believe possible. And that we will *always* underestimate that capacity.

I have tried to give a conception of this size by using the ocean and beaches analogy. But the analogy also shows how the vast bulk of what is in our minds lies hidden and unseen, and how only a tiny part of it can ever appear on the surface at one time. So that is the first explanation: we can do more things than we think we can because the capacity of our minds is larger than we assume – larger than we believe possible.

I said they were going to be simple.

Explanation 2 Interval training

Another commonplace observation which we ignore because we think it can't be true is that skills improve in the *intervals* between practices. We are so indoctrinated with the message that it is only the hard work of constant and unremitting practice which can bring improvement and success that we discount the little voice inside us which says, 'I think my tennis serve is better at the beginning of this season than it was at the end of the last.'

'Shhh you fool, it can't be', we say. But once we get into the habit of listening to these little nudges from our subconscious we find that they are surprisingly reliable guides.

Then we can set about thinking of explanations. One may be that the patterns of co-ordination and control sort themselves out over time and emerge simplified and clarified in some subtle way which is inhibited if we bash on with relentless practice.

Or, because our minds telescope memories of one category of things by collecting them up in the same memory box, we get far more expert through occasional practice than would be expected when we see the events in their literal context. Our total experience of a particular skill, although spread over a long period, is often substantial. And, quite automatically, our minds do exactly what is necessary to maximize the benefit from this distributed experience. They collect it all together in the same box and exclude other things from our attention.

This is how I discovered 'Willis' sign for malaria – a small thing but mine own. Willis' sign for malaria is positive when the patient walks into the room and says 'I've got malaria!' For the six cases of malaria I have seen during my career I have found it to be an infallible guide. It works because patients with malaria always know they've been exposed and haven't been taking their prophylaxis, or they have had it before. To make this important medical discovery my mind must have selected a rule which all six of my cases, distributed over twenty years or so, had in common. No mean achievement, but quite automatic. All the thousands upon thousands of other disease categories which would have confused the picture and prevented me seeing a pattern were excluded from the 'malaria' box.

Explanation 3 The law of multiple returns

Many things in life conform to the 'law of diminishing returns'. It says that things are easy at first and get more and more difficult as you progress. Like all laws it isn't entirely true, but it is a useful model of why it is hard to do things well, and next to impossible to do them *best*. I would like to look at it the other way round, as one of nature's gifts to those who do things in general. Here is what I mean.

During the past ten years or so the 'jogging' craze has taught a whole generation of adults the previously unsuspected fact that with a minimum of preparation any normally healthy individual can sustain a jog-trot for as long as it takes boredom to overtake them.

All you have to do to get the maximum return for your training effort, with the minimum risk of giving up because of strains and other injuries, is about twenty minutes, three times a week. This is the same for any other sustained, vigorous exercise. Much less, I believe, than most people would have expected.

Compare this with the training programme needed to succeed in competition. It is clear that a great many other things can be done with the time and energy difference, especially since a moderate amount of exercise actually *increases* your total energy and vitality. So provided you *do* do other things as well, each at a moderate level, you will obtain a far greater total return of benefit than if you had applied the same amount of energy all on one thing. (But only you will be in a position to judge. Other people will insist on measuring your success by a single parameter!)

The important thing is to know what your objective is. If you want to be the best in the world in some field, and in our present culture many people do, then you have no alternative but to try to exert yourself with greater dedication than anybody else. If you have natural ability of course it helps, but in most fields there will be plenty of people with natural ability.

Single-minded devotion to training has been the common factor necessary for success in numerous competitive activities throughout the latter part of this century. There has been a runaway escalation of training schedules which must certainly have prejudiced other aspects of the development of the individuals involved.

This is bad enough for the few who are successful, whom we hear about, but what about the many who are not and whom we do not hear about? Nobody wants to read stories about people who devote all the daylight hours of their childhoods to perfecting their butterfly stroke only to fail to achieve success.

The alternative objective, which is currently unfashionable, is to be a well rounded, well balanced, broadly educated and complete human being. A so-called 'renaissance man'. This sort of person can justifiably enjoy the enormous achievement of coming *last* in the London Marathon. For this sort of person the law of diminishing returns is transformed into the law of multiple returns.

Explanation 4 The power of analogy

It is a truly extraordinary fact that we can apply the same delicacy and control with which we steer a car along a winding road to handling a difficult interview with an estranged couple. This is another example of the enormously significant and powerful mechanism of analogy.

In our minds all the different things we do are in one sense separate and in another sense make-up one 'whole'. Every single thing in our minds merges into this mysterious continuum. This enables our minds to perform a feat which would be an imposs- ible dream for the designers of computers who are restricted to finite units of information. Our minds express everything relative to everything else. Almost any pair of concepts, however ridicu- lously dissimilar, are scrutinized automatically and common fea- tures found. Incredibly, these common features are then used for a mutual enhancement of *both* the original concepts. This mechanism is exactly what is needed to simplify the task of handling the real world. Everything is dealt with by analogy.

Even when we approach a new task for the first time we begin with a complete set of behaviour patterns which our mind has selected as being most nearly like what it expects the new task to be. This match is often extremely good and even if it isn't the mind instantly begins to improve it in the light of experience, using other existing patterns as it does so.

Thus practically any skill, and any knowledge, is relevant to practically anything else.

The fact that we cannot understand how this happens, that we cannot understand how it could happen, that we couldn't begin to make a machine to imitate it happening, doesn't alter the fact that it *does* happen. All you have to do to prove that it happens is to notice it doing so.

I have no doubt that many of the skills I develop doing things like mending a lock, digging the garden, sailing a boat, acting as a governor at a local school, singing, or even sitting doing nothing on a summer day, are applicable to making me a better doctor. Or a better father, or husband. Somehow it seems obvious and trite to point such things out. But something is happening to our society which makes it necessary to do so.

Explanation 5 The pump priming effect

Perhaps the most obvious of these explanations is the pump-priming effect. This is the burden of well-known sayings such as 'Things that can be done at any time are never done at all', and 'If you want something done, get someone who is busy to do it.'

We all know that we are more efficient when something has already got us going. All sorts of jobs get done in a flash once we have got into the swing of things. We develop a momentum and it seems almost effortless just to feed a few extra tasks through the whirling machinery, even when those tasks might have been quite daunting in isolation.

At other times, when we are dull and unmotivated, we get nothing done at all. As my friend and colleague Christopher Everett once pointed out, the thing that takes longest about gardening is getting out of your chair. This same effect is the explanation for the surprising but common experience of doctors that they get most behind time in surgery when they are *not* under pressure. Once again the surprise is an unerring pointer to the significance. You may well share the surprise, but the observation is true.

Explanation 6 Motivation

Just as in the example of jogging, the emphasis on competitiveness and success in the present-day world has led to the tragic belief that something is only worth doing if it can be done successfully. In other words, if it can be done better than other people can do it. To make matters worse, people make their judgement of success on the media scale.

A beneficial side-effect of this has been what is almost certainly a general increase in the standards of performance in numerous fields as people emulate the international superstars. But much of this benefit is off-set by people being made to realize how second-rate their performances are and then wondering whether it is worth the effort.

The word 'amateur' of course comes from the Latin verb '*amo, I love*'. An amateur does things for the love of them. As so often happens, the original meaning of a word holds the key to understanding. Do things for the sheer joy of them. Do lots of things. Do them as well as you can, of course, but judge that against your own standards, not some impossible standards set by somebody else.

In case this heresy should be causing too much distress I must qualify it. First by saying that this approach does not exclude the high-flyer from going off down the competitive road. The two approaches are complementary. On the other hand, if the specialist sportsman is finding that his training has become so all-consuming that his life is becoming distorted and narrow, I do think that he should re-examine his values. Certainly those of us who look on from the terraces should have the courage to question those values and not to go on unthinkingly admiring them.

Once again let me emphasize that the reason I am not arguing the case for the pursuit of excellence is not because I don't think it is a good case. Quite the reverse. The case is so strong and so central to the present day ethos of the world that it does not *need* arguing. What I am seeking is a healthy *balance* and to achieve that I must argue the opposing case which is so sadly neglected.

Explanation 7 Skimming the cream

People often say to me, 'You must spend an awful lot of time keeping up to date!'

In a sense I do. I see about a dozen medical journals a week, I attend clinical meetings, I discuss diagnoses and treatments with specialists, I continually look up facts in reference books, etc.

The idea that there are dozens of new advances in medicine which are constantly changing everything is a myth however.

The important advances in medicine which are likely to be of relevance to a general practitioner in caring for his patients can usually be read in the columns, if not the headlines, of a respons- ible newspaper. Not only that, but the news of major advances is invariably repeated over and over again in different places.

The main truths of any other discipline can also be obtained relatively simply. This is certainly not to deny the enormous complexity of the knowledge base that is required to understand any particular field at the level you need to contribute to advances in that field. These two things are quite different.

The fact is that when it comes to getting the cream of vital ideas from any specialist field, nature favours the generalist. He can gallop about plundering innumerable fields for their best ideas. Ideas like those of Leonardo da Vinci and Popper and Einstein, which required genius, inspiration, luck and ency- clopaedic knowledge of the accumulated ideas of mankind for their origin, are there to be used by everybody else. It may not seem fair, but it is true, and we are very foolish if we do not make use of this fact. In doing so we come to respect the original thinkers even more but that is only incidental.

Maintaining a broad knowledge base

Those of us who are fortunate enough to live in the developed world now have a greater freedom of access to the collected knowledge of mankind than any people in history. The selective power of our minds, which evolved in response to the pressures of a very different world, is serving us astonishingly well in making sense of the deluge of information brought to us by technology.

Not only are we exposed to newspapers, books, periodicals, radio, television, films, computer databases, but to educational organizations and techniques of unprecedented refinement and availability. There has never been a time when there were more fascinating and important things going on in the world or when they were better presented to be accessible to the understanding of ordinary people. It would be a terrible irony if this unpre- cedented situation were to coincide with a general feeling that people should not attempt to dabble in specialist fields.

From my perspective as a doctor I have no doubt whatever

that dabbling, or skimming the cream, is entirely legitimate. Provided we are honest with ourselves and with each other. The important thing is to know our limitations. It is far more important for a doctor to know his limitations than it is for him to be terribly clever. Throughout life, being honest is utterly fundamental.

But not only is dabbling legitimate, it is a responsibility, and one which we all share. In the future, more and more of the effort of life is inevitably going to be directed to maintaining the artificial systems, technological and organizational, which make our lives possible. But the hidden oceans formed by the complex ideas which underpin society are held in a form which, although it appears to be sophisticated, is ludicrously primitive when compared with the way in which ideas are held in our own minds. In particular, information technology is nowhere near providing any sort of equivalent for the automatic mechanisms which continually scrutinize the oceans of ideas in our minds for incongruities.

Everything in nature happens for a reason and if we don't imitate these natural scrutinizing processes we will inevitably find out their importance by bitter experience. But maintaining the whole is an unimaginably larger job than watching the frothy fringes upon which society focuses its collective attention. There is only one conceivable way in which we can hope to cope with this huge task and that is to devolve it to the common sense of individual people.

The world will only continue to work if people keep in touch with the breadth of human knowledge at the same time as they pursue their narrow specialist fields. In other words, if we wish to participate in a democracy we must all accept responsibility for educating our common sense.

To do this we have to be able to rely on the information which we skim. And although our minds boggle at the apparent sophistication of contemporary technology for storing, manipulating and communicating information we sometimes forget the simple fact that the whole edifice of information technology is valueless unless the information stored, manipulated and communicated is true.

The answer to everything

Life is always more complicated than we think it is. We will always underestimate the hidden background to the things that we see on the surface. And that seems, on the face of it, to be a justification for the specialist approach and for the formal scientific method. In other words; if everything is so complicated there is no point in trying to cope with it all and the only possible way forward is by logical reduction and by specialization.

It is absolutely essential that we try to cope with the general background. In order to do so we have to accept that this can only be achieved as an approximation, it cannot be precise and perfect. Although this sort of approach is diametrically opposed to the convergent, materialistic, mechanistic, specialized approach, that does not mean that one is 'good' and the other is 'bad'. Both are necessary. Both must be kept in balance with each other. And there is no way of achieving this balance in a precise, defined, analysed and formally justifiable way. The only way of doing it is by using the profoundly mysterious abilities of the human mind.

So although it is in a sense easier to be a specialist, to choose one mountain and then climb it all the way to the top, the job of being a generalist, who gets to know a little of every mountain, is ultimately the more important one. Specialization is a tool just as language is a tool. Both are immensely powerful and important tools which we should all use but they are not essential to life. The forming of a general, overall, self-consistent image of the world *is* essential to life. If, through our failure to appreciate the importance and the sheer difficulty of that task, we undervalue it and attempt to abdicate it to machines and externally imposed rules of society we will find life progressively impoverished just when we think we are making the greatest progress.

Many people feel that that is exactly what is happening today.

11

Good intentions

In its fervour to put right imperfections in the world, society has ensnared its members in a web of regulations which create new problems and diminish life.

'How long since you had your last baby?'
'Four years.'
'Oh *well*! They've changed it *all* since then!'
Auxiliary nurse in a postnatal ward, officiously telling a mother how to change the nappy of her fourth baby.

Throughout this book, I have used my experience of general practice as an analogy for life in a technological world. I have tried to show how personal relationships between individual people provide us with the 'why' of life whereas technology can only ever provide us with the 'how'. And I have given, I hope, some explanations for our common experience that we can cope with the complexity of modern life far better than either instinct or formal logic would lead us to expect. It remains to summarize the symptoms of our ailing technological society. Then I can make a diagnosis, and finally write my prescription.

I have puzzled over how to encapsulate the problem in a useful way. Most people will acknowledge that the great bell of Progress which rang throughout the post-war years has developed a cracked sound. I could fill chapters with examples which nobody would have time or inclination to read. So, once again,

I think it will be best to give just a little of the flavour. Something that happened last week is fresh in my memory . . .

'It's progress, isn't it'

I'm on a call-out to a new block of sheltered flats. In spite of the sales office flags the place has a slightly desolate air as quite a few of the units are still unsold. This is due to the slump in the housing market, not to a shortage of elderly people. Plenty of spaces for cars, anyway, and I draw up right outside the front door. I find number twenty-five on the bank of call buttons, press once and peer expectantly at the little grill, watching for a voice. Sure enough, before long the grill crackles and says:

> 'Hello.'
>
> 'It's Dr Willis . . .'
>
> 'Oh. OK, Doctor. I'll release the door for you.'

I turn to look at the door catch and listen for the click. Nothing happens. I try the door. Firm as a rock. I wait. I sigh. I press the bell again.

A head pops out of a second floor window fifty yards behind me.

> 'Hasn't it worked, Doctor?'
>
> 'No', I shout.
>
> 'OK, I'll come down.'

I wait again. Looking idly at the bank of buttons, neatly machined out of a metal plate. As it has just the right number of buttons it must have been designed and made specially. Then I notice that one of the buttons is different. Instead of having a room number, it had a letter 'T' on it. I have the amusing idea that it might be a 'Test' button which would bypass all the security arrangements and open the door straight away. My finger is drawn towards it mischievously. Then I decide that such a thing would be ridiculous and I'd be much more likely to trigger some sort of embarrassing security alert. Better wait.

Through the glass front door I watch the lights on the lift control panel across the hall until they tell me that my patient has successfully negotiated the second floor corridor and is on his way down. The call was for a giddy turn, so this is useful diagnostic information. The lights change as they follow the slow descent of the lift and at last the doors open. I watch with relief as he steadily crosses the hall towards me, smiling in his familiar, apologetic way. Most of the nastier explanations of the giddiness melt away. This is going to be a pleasant, mainly social call. Very different from six months before when he had been waiting for me at the entrance, anxious to hurry me up to where his wife lay on her bed, desperately ill after a sudden stroke and never to regain consciousness.

> 'I'm sorry you had to come down but it didn't seem to work at all.'

We look resentfully at the mechanism and I mention my discovery:

> 'There's a button here marked "T". It couldn't mean "Test", could it?'

> 'Oh, no. I think that's the one for tradesmen.'

> 'I don't believe it! Let's try.'

I pop outside again, close the door and press the 'T'. The latch clicks back instantly and I walk back in. Silly of me not to have tried . . . On the way up to the flat we agree that it is a good thing you can trust tradesmen.

When I have checked him over I reassure him about the giddy turn. He seems fine.

> 'I didn't want to call you myself, but the warden said she had to. It's in the rules, apparently.'

I look up from writing in the notes:

> 'Sorry, I don't understand. What do you mean, she had to?'

'She says, any call she gets she has to fill in a form and say she has called the doctor.'

'But that's crazy. What does she *do* with the form? Who reads it? How are they to know what was the right thing to do? They are just people, like you and me. Why can't they just let her use her common sense?'

'I know, Doctor, I know. It's completely crackers.'

'But what are we going to *do* about it? The world is going completely mad.'

'But there's nothing you *can* do.' He laughs, 'It's progress, isn't it.'

Teachers

My wife has been a teacher as long as I have been a doctor. So, what with the friends and patients who are teachers, my own experience at various levels of medical education, and my experience as a college governor, I do know something about education. For example, I know that teachers are just as frustrated and demoralized as doctors are by progress.

Apparently, one of the chores in the life of a teacher is constructing tables of so-called rank orders. What you do is to apply a formula to all the marks you have available for each pupil and you end up with an overall figure which enables you to put them into an order. Now, the interesting thing my wife has noticed is that although you know as the teacher that the individual marks you use to arrive at the result are all approximations, once you have given each pupil their rank it is almost impossible not to think of them in that order from then on. The figure, however arbitrary, always takes precedence over the feeling, even in the mind that originated both. If Jennifer came one place ahead of Jean, you cannot stop yourself thinking she is 'better' than Jean.

Now whole schools are to be given rank orders and the means by which they are derived are even more arbitrary. But here again, the figure is the thing that counts, and comes to take precedence over the subtle and balanced view of traditional common sense. And here again, it is next to impossible to articulate the passionate conviction of experienced teachers that the new measurements are naive and damaging. Their pleas that rigid job descriptions and contracts and assessments and audits and mission statements are all two-edged weapons which can be profoundly detrimental to the professional values and motivation that have served mankind throughout history go largely unheard. It is not just in the modern BBC that respected seniors are dismissed contemptuously as being 'tainted by experience'; I know that teachers of exactly the kind that you and I would wish to have educating our children feel that their experience is held in contempt by the new system. I know because they tell me so in surgery when they ask me to support their requests for early retirement.

Nurses

I couldn't help laughing as I walked into our beautiful new GP ward recently and found the sister and two staff nurses buried in paperwork which completely covered the surfaces of their smart new nursing station.

'A picture of modern nursing', I said.
They looked up, genuinely surprised.

'Is that the impression it gives?'

'Yes, it is!'

It takes fifteen A4 sheets (prettily colour-coded) to admit a patient to our ward these days and so far from being seen as a problem by the managers, this system has actually won a prize. People really do believe that this sort of thing is progress.

Within a week of a widely publicized baby snatch from a maternity unit in the Midlands (and before the baby had been restored to an anxious nation) all these nurses, some of whom we have worked with for twenty years, sprouted ID badges complete with photographs, like a lot of operatives in a nuclear arsenal. This of course was a knee-jerk reaction by the administrators – any would-be baby snatcher would have a hard time of it on our ward, or indeed in any hospital within fifteen miles, because there aren't any babies. Any grannies that they snatched would probably enjoy the outing. Meanwhile the message those dreadful badges give about the kind of organization the ward has become, and the state of the society it exists in, is being received, loud and clear, by every visitor every day of the week.

I remember my astonishment when the midwife who works with our practice was sent away on a two week course in stitching, leaving all her devoted patients in the hands of a series of stand-ins. Stitching is strictly part of the doctor's job but in the old, living world she had been doing it as well if not better than any of us for, we worked out, well over ten years. In the new rigid world she was suddenly told that she couldn't stitch because she hadn't been on the necessary course and she hadn't got the right certificate. So, unbelievably, she was taken off duties for two weeks so that she could be trained 'properly'. Although it was obvious to everybody that the rules were crazy, nobody had the authority to use their common sense and overrule them.

We seem to be approaching the point at which nobody can do anything unless they have been trained and assessed in it. But although having been trained in something appears to be a proof that you can do it well, common sense tells us that there is much more to it than that. Ordinary people can very easily conceive of the possibility that a training course might actually make somebody *less* good at something. Being a sympathetic listener is perhaps a clearer example than stitching. But people running courses on sympathetic listening, or on stitching, are not acting as ordinary people, they are acting as experts. What's more they have a vested interest in promoting the cult of training. Training totally ignores the most vital component of performance, motivation. Training is all about 'How?' Never about 'Why?'

It was a bitter and certainly unintentional irony that the new system which has so massively increased the paperwork in modern nursing, imported from America even as it was wisely being abandoned there, was called The Nursing Process. As a result of this innovation, nurses have joined the ranks of all those other people in the modern world who spend huge chunks of their time filling in standard procedure sheets. In theory it sounds a good idea to structure and define the job and record how it is done. It seems that it must result in a better service. It will enable managers to count the items of service and prove how much has been done. But you only have to talk to patients to find out the result, they say those poor nurses are too busy to talk to them. It's common sense again. Process is pure how. Nature cries out that nursing is predominantly why.

Doctors

General practitioners are a bunch of individualists, perhaps the last professional generalists, impossible to deal with as a group but useful to have around when you need them. It cannot be overemphasized how profoundly the growth of central control and management technology threatens their traditional role. For a traditional role it is – there is an ecological niche for something of the kind in virtually all societies and at every point in history. But now the clash of cultures appears to be irreconcilable.

The technological society has problems with any form of individualism, but in a field as serious as medicine it is obviously completely intolerable. Individualists working within the bright new machine would prove that it wasn't perfect, because they clearly couldn't all be right at once. Dangerously free agents, GPs have operated out of control for too long. They need a good dose of 'progress' to bring them into line. They won't like it, of course, but it will do them good ... As Jaques Ellul predicted half a century ago in *The Technological Society*, 'Mankind is to be smoothed out, like a pair of trousers under a steam iron.'

There is now a crisis of morale in the medical profession which mirrors that in other professions, and although I could see it coming, it has largely materialized since 1984 when I began to work on the project which has become this book. At that time, when medicine itself was the most popular career for bright school-leavers, general practice was the number one career choice for British doctors. We really were getting the cream of the nation's youth.

Something terrible has happened since then. Nobody wants to go into general practice any more and all the established doctors can't wait to get out. Everybody says the same thing – there is too much paperwork, we have lost our independence, and the pressures get more and more unbearable. We seem to have been taken over by the same alien culture that we have seen spreading throughout the rest of modern society.

THE NEW CULTURE

- How? (*process*) rather than why? (*purpose*).
- Specialism (*exclusion*) rather than generalism (*inclusion*).
- Blind rule-following rather than action based on understanding.
- Training rather than education.
- External, imposed motivation rather than personal and internal.
- Corporate rather than individual responsibility.
- Certainty rather than risk-taking.
- Attention to measurable parts rather than indefinable wholes.
- Attention to surface appearance rather than hidden depth and content.
- Rigid mechanism rather than the flexibility and diversity of nature.

Part of the problem is that we are entering a new phase of medicine which is inherently less satisfying for doctors, in which illnesses really are much less common and are caught at a stage when they are in fact much less troublesome.

It's a bit like the worry I used to have as a young idealist that if we solved all the problems of the world there would be nothing left to live for. I soon realized that solving all the problems of the world was not an immediate prospect, but doctors do get most of their satisfaction and motivation in life from finding illnesses and making people better and it is true that the more successful they are at the preventative side of their work and the more they find illnesses before the patients feel they have got anything wrong with them, the less they get this vital buzz.

So, contrary to what might have been expected, medical progress has not resulted in masses of grateful patients thanking doctors for the blessing of good health. On the contrary, not only do patients tend to feel that they have a right to be well, and that if something is wrong with them it is somebody's fault, but they also tend to take treatments somewhat resentfully because they haven't got any symptoms yet. As Osler said, 'It is hard to make someone who feels well, feel better.'

Instead they become irrationally obsessed with fashionable media scares and are intolerant of any side effects or dangers of their treatment. Persuading patients to take their medicine is now a very significant problem indeed. Hardly a week goes by without someone bringing in a newspaper scare story or a warning sheet issued by a litigation-wary pharmacist and sheepishly saying that they've stopped taking their treatment because of the warnings. The days when patients would say, 'Give me something really *strong*, Doctor, it's kill or cure, isn't it!' are now quite gone, although I can certainly remember them. Today such blind trust is only bestowed on the herbalist. Never mind, moves are afoot to get them to issue warning sheets as well.

Pushing against a spring

There is another demoralizing effect as doctors are required by society to behave more and more perfectly and to be more and more infallible. Everything is getting more difficult as we get nearer and nearer to perfection. However high our standards, people will come to judge our performance by those standards – regardless of the difficulty of maintaining them. The nearer we get to achieving this impossible ideal the more we feel that we are subject to criticism and feelings of inadequacy. When we push forward to a new balance point at which our available energy is matched by a new, higher level of complexity, any errors that we then make will be just as prominent as the errors which we made previously at what was actually a lower level of effort and complexity. It is like pushing against a spring.

The importance of errors is another thing which is assessed relatively not absolutely. In absolute terms, the old errors were actually more important because they occurred at a lower level of perfection. (When I started in my present practice I had no less than three patients whose lives had been blighted by botched thyroid operations – all by the same surgeon – two of them had silver tracheostomy tubes in their throats for the rest of their lives and the third was permanently hoarse.) But because the things that are now being attempted are inherently nearer to an impossible level of perfection, it appears that *more* errors are being made and that the service is getting *worse*, not better as is actually the case.

Medicine has never been safer than it is today, yet public anxiety about safety has never been higher. Although we have made enormous progress, society's appetite for further progress and ever greater levels of safety seems impossible to satisfy.

Regulation

It is in response to this situation that the present vogue for centralized decision-making and regulation has arisen. It is an inescapable fact that the first reaction to any tragedy such as the baby snatch already referred to is to look around for somebody to blame. Strangely enough this person rarely seems to be the person who snatched the baby. The automatic response of the all-powerful media commentators is to look for more regulation. Time and again you hear them talking as if more and better regulations can only be a good thing.

No matter that the hospital concerned had only just had a security review and already had a department of specialist security officers and, who knows, perhaps even ID badges for its nurses; a junior minister was wheeled on to say that he was going to make sure security was tightened even further! And I can tell him something – the rarer such incidents become, the *more* will be the outrage, the anger and the calls for further controls. Poor chap, even Hercules might have quailed at such a labour!

And, er, the baby was, let me remind you, returned. But oh, so much less boring than the five (or is it seven) people killed each day on the roads!

The futile attempt to live to a standard which will eliminate media scale risks is destroying the joy of life for individual people living in the real world. Risks which are only perceptible on the media scale can only be prevented by media scale supervision, and that leaves little role for the individual. Often the minuscule good done by the elimination of a remote, theoretical risk is outweighed many times by the harm done to the independence and motivation of people.

But that doesn't worry the regulators in the least. They have all the certainty that they are right of converts to a new religion. They are absolutely unshakable in their conviction that the representation of everything in rigid rules and formal mathematical models is the very epitome of progress and they present their beliefs with a self-confidence, not to say arrogance, which would be fatuous if it were not so familiar.

Speaking their own strange language, they talk of attempting to *'capture'* the problems we front line workers are desperately trying to get them to understand. The shortage of community nurses is a recent example:

> 'We are trying to *map* the nursing services in your area.'

> 'Yes, but we are all busy people who have come here to tell you that the shortages are our top priority!'

> 'Ah yes, but we have got to have the *data* to make a *proper business case.'*

Notice the implications of the word 'proper'.

> 'Look, the nurses have been using their computers to make their returns for years – where is all *that* data?'

They look at us primitives with pitying eyes.

The trouble is that we have broken the feedback loop. The people who make decisions are no longer the ones who see what happens as a result. They don't think they need to because they are so sure that their models are a much more accurate, reliable and valid way of finding out what is happening. They completely reject the old way of doing things, which is to let the vast bulk of the world sink into the ocean of congruity and just concentrate on the problems that appear on the surface of the mind. By wildly underestimating the size, complexity and subtlety of the ocean that they are dealing with, they think it is a huge advance to use their new machines to model the whole thing at once.

What we have here is an uncontrolled experiment, which looks as if it is going to be an historic failure. You have to make an effort to remind yourself that these ideas, which have overturned the means by which mankind has made progress since the dawn of civilization, have been current for little more than ten years.

It is the replacement of individual experience, common sense, and responsibility by an external structure of rules which is the key change in the new situation. Although originally created by us, this structure of rules has now taken on an existence which

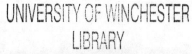

is quite independent of any single human mind. The tools we originally created to serve our needs have taken over and made us their servants.

The impracticality of strict adherence to rules as a way of running the world is a matter of common sense. In industry the term 'working to rule' actually means the same as going on strike. But when any of us looks at the world from a restricted view point we can't avoid the distortions of perception. Doctors are notorious for not following their own rules when they take medicines and I sometimes think that anyone who can take tablets four times a day without fail is an obsessional neurotic and probably needs treatment for that. Nonetheless, we go on expecting people to do it. When I started work at the Middlesex Hospital my senior medical registrar told me that our job in life was to make sure the patients died with their electrolytes balanced (in other words having the right proportions of sodium and potassium salts in their blood). Once, I commented to a local undertaker on a body lying rosy-cheeked in his chapel – 'He looks surprisingly well, considering he's dead!'

Joking apart, when doctors work to rule there is a grave danger that the rules will do better than the patients.

Balance and unbalance

I remember visiting an old lady when I first started in my present practice. She wanted something new for her aching knees and I gave her my honest, scientific doctor's advice, according to the rules. I said that she had already tried everything that could conceivably be of any value, from every sort of painkilling and anti-inflammatory drug to bandages, rubbing creams and physiotherapy and that there was really nothing more that could be done. I was very sorry but the Paracetamol she was already having were as effective as anything else, safer and cheaper and that I thought she should go on taking them.

There was a pause and she surveyed me shrewdly. 'You know,' she said, 'Dr Larcombe (my predecessor) would never have said that. He knew it wouldn't really make any difference and I knew that it wouldn't, but he always gave me something.'

Then more kindly, 'You're young though – you'll learn.'

Over the years I have told this story to a number of doctors who remain completely unmoved by it and go on insisting that I was right in the blunt truth which I gave. But I have no doubt at all that the old lady was right. At the same time I continue to believe that modern medicine is founded on the bedrock of science and that to abandon science would be to return to the dark ages. These two approaches may seem to be opposites when we view them literally and scientifically but our minds possess the mysterious artistry necessary to merge the two opposites into a balanced synthesis and a way forward.

Long after that old lady died scientific evidence began to accumulate which has now proved beyond reasonable doubt that virtually any treatment which a patient believes in will indeed help them, physically and measurably. This means that science has proved that doctors can always help patients who trust them. Which is what the old lady knew all along!

Diagnosis

We use the word 'unbalanced' to describe an insane mind. Thus the accumulated wisdom embodied in the very language we speak acknowledges the fundamental role of balance in the definition of sanity. So when I say that the common mind of our society is unbalanced, I am making a very serious diagnosis. I am saying that the common mind of society is, to some extent, insane. But that is what I do say.

The overwhelming tendency in the modern world is to listen to the hard, precisely-defined certainties of the expert and to disregard the softer, more vulnerable, but far more important balanced hypothesis of the generalist. As a result, very many aspects of the contemporary world which seem logical and sensible when viewed in isolation by the remote specialists who are in charge of them, seem obvious madness to everybody else.

The current trend towards external review of everything is fundamentally flawed. The idea that regulation is a good thing *per se* is an illusion. Regulation destroys humanity. It undervalues the individual human being, his mind, his motivation and his integrity. Unfortunately GPs have to some extent colluded in the process of reducing their practice to a lot of sterile formulae. They have done this because they have shared in the illusion that this is what is necessary for progress. This means that general practice, the last great bastion of professional generalism and common sense, is being judged by the wrong criteria. It has lost its self-respect because it is trying to express itself in a language which denies its very nature.

> 'There's nothing you *can* do about it, doctor, it's progress isn't it!'

Fortunately he hadn't been too giddy to get to the front door to let me in, and he certainly wasn't unbalanced, but I didn't agree with him. Sitting on the nice, comfortable sofa in the flat that he had hoped to share for much longer with his wife, I told him that I thought there *was* something we could do about it.

12

Prescription

As society becomes more technologically sophisticated it becomes more and more essential that individual members do not abdicate their common sense and their integrity.

'Will it sting?'
'Well, it might sting a bit, but you won't mind too much.'
'Well, actually, I would mind if it stings.'
Five year old being prescribed eye drops.

'I think he's dead, doctor'

The veins in the big farmer's arm stand out like ropes and the needle goes in easily. I release the tourniquet and begin to inject the Diamorphine, a tenth of a millilitre at a time, watching the tension, the pain and the sweat in his face. I listen to his breathing, feeling his pulse with my free hand. I feel rather alone at the end of the long road and the rough farm track.

'You'll feel better in a moment . . . Don't worry . . .'

He opens his eyes and smiles a little.

'Any different?'

'It's easing off a bit, I think.'

'OK. Just rest back . . .'

I watch and wait for him to settle. Holding back half the syringe.

'Could we have a bowl in case he feels sick please.'

His wife goes out briskly.

It is my weekend on duty and they are patients of one of the other doctors in the rota. It sounded like a coronary on the telephone and when I arrived it looked like one. It obviously felt like one.

I'm thinking what to do next. Whether to admit him to hospital or keep him at home. I decide to be frank with him. He's no fool, he'll want to know.

'Now I think what's happened is that you've had a slight . . . Hang on . . . Damn!'

He's not listening. His eyes are rolling upwards. Even as my hands go to lift his chin he takes a convulsive unconscious inspiration, stops breathing and begins to turn blue.

This is not my favourite pastime . . . I slap the centre of his chest hard – worked once, but not this time. I make a space and swing his heavy body on to the floor, stick a plastic airway from my emergency bag over his tongue and begin to inflate his chest with my Ambu-bag. There is no pulse – so I start cardiac massage as well. His wife is looking on. What do I do next?

I remember suddenly my colleague who is on duty for the other practice and who I know has a defibrillator in his car which we might use to get the farmer's heart beating again.

'Look, could you ring this number and ask Dr Bethell to get here as quickly as possible.'

I know it is stupid as I say it. He couldn't possibly be here in less than twenty minutes and we haven't a hope of saving him after more than five. She goes off anyway and I draw up some Adrenaline and inject it into his heart. Nothing. He is turning bluer so I go back to the respiration and the cardiac massage knowing that I am only doing it because I haven't the courage to stop.

And then I feel the gentle touch on my shoulder and the soft voice of his wife, trying not to upset me too much;

> 'I think he's dead, doctor . . .'

Allowed to use my common sense

I know that lady well now because she came on to my own list of patients when my colleague retired. After her husband's death she left the farm and moved to a smaller house. Now she keeps her new garden as full of brilliant flowers as she used to keep the old one. After the night of the great storm of October 1987 she told me that she had lain there, alone in her bedroom, hearing the trees crashing down on to her lawn, one after another. She said:

> 'I thought the end of the world had come. I didn't mind very much, I just lay there and waited.'

You don't need to tell me the number of different ways I could have treated her husband better, how much better equipped I could have been or how much better trained for that particular eventuality. Nobody could have felt these deficiencies more than I did. But her straightforward common sense brought home to me just how irrelevant, how intrusive and how trivial such hi-tec interventions would actually have been.

There is no correct answer to the problem of how far to push the treatment of dying patients, the only answer is common sense. That's why heads of state get such an appalling deal at the ends of their lives. Teams of the most distinguished doctors available are assembled and while the whole world watches in horror they struggle to prevent what is obviously inevitable.

Nobody, however senior or distinguished, can afford to be guided by common sense when their actions are spotlighted on the media stage. So Emperor Hirohito of Japan, President Eisenhower of the USA and General Franco of Spain went through days and weeks of unnecessary suffering because nobody had the courage to say the simple words, 'I think he's dying, doctor.'

When I die I hope that I will have a doctor who is free to use his, or her, common sense. I know from numerous remarks made to me by patients over the years that this is what other people want as well: to be able to trust a doctor to weigh up the situation and treat them as they would treat a member of their own family. No more. No less. Most people are far more afraid of too much treatment at the end of their lives than of too little and few expect their doctors to go on saving them for ever. But they do expect them to use their common sense. It is vital that we create a society which can respect such final wishes of its members.

What role for the individual?

I have tried to give some impression in this book of the wonderful cast of characters that peoples the world of one small-town GP. I have quoted some of the things they say in order to show the wisdom, love and humanity of ordinary people, which the media phenomenon has somehow misled us into doubting.

It is individual people who are important in life, with their infinite variations, colours, strengths and failures. Yet, more and more, people are asking what role there is for them as individuals in the impersonal, mechanistic society they increasingly live in. They feel that there must be more to life than just being an anonymous operative in a great machine, or an anonymous consumer, whose actions can be reduced to a series of statistical norms.

What I have tried to do is to go beyond the simple statement of an inner conviction. To express more than 'just a feeling' that without the human aspects of life, life would not be worth living. I have set out to show that there are excellent, logical reasons why society needs the common sense and integrity of individual people in order to sort out the tangle of proliferating technology that enmeshes us. After we have dealt with the cold logic of the matter, those who want to put the feelings back in again are free to join me in doing so.

The crux of the paradox

Here we are at the crux of the paradox. We want to define clear solutions to the problems we can see in the world. But as we do so we progressively destroy the essence of life itself. It seems to be an unavoidable rule that the precise definition of human affairs has the effect of killing humanity itself.

To put it another way, society is faced with the following problem; we understand the world we live in more completely than we have ever done before, and yet we understand it less. The near total triumph of our logical approach to quantifying and measuring and recording the world looks like coinciding with our final destruction, by one means or another, of that world. In other words, our logical approach to life is threatening to bring our life to a logical conclusion. And the irony is that our slide into the abyss will be understood and explained and recorded like the greatest cinema epic there has ever been.

As Robert M Pirsig said in his wonderful book, *Zen and the Art of Motorcycle Maintenance*, '. . . the crisis is being caused by the inadequacy of existing forms of thought to cope with the situation. It can't be solved by rational means because the rationality itself is the source of the problem.'

As we hunt, more and more frantically, for ways to describe and control the world more and more perfectly, we find that the problems don't get less, they get more. Daily, we encounter the consequences of our failed perception. And all the time the answer we are seeking is there, not actually under our noses, but an inch or two above and behind our noses.

Our minds

I don't want to get involved in the familiar argument about whether or not our minds are machines. There can be no question that our minds have qualities of subtlety and mystery which place them far beyond our normal conception of what is meant by a machine. Whether the capacities for self-awareness, passion and free will are ultimately explainable in solely mechanistic terms is beyond me, although I have my view. But what I would say is that if our capacity for understanding – this amazing ability which we take so much for granted – to hold an imaginary model of the world, to constantly improve it by comparison with experience, and then by applying something which we call imagination, to test out future courses of action and future possible developments – if this ability is the function of a machine, that machine is like no machine that man has ever created.

The modern assumption is that we have machines and systems which describe and therefore understand the world better than our minds could ever do. We assume that we have improved enormously on nature. But we are entirely wrong. Not only have we underestimated the magnitude of the task we have undertaken, not only have we failed to appreciate the power of our minds, but we have failed to see that the absolute terms in which machines are compelled to operate are incapable of describing life *at all*.

Machines are in their element when dealing with absolute terms; they are enormously superior to us at, for example, performing calculations. Computers, after all, compute. But when we extrapolate from this, as many people do, to the assumption that they will be correspondingly superior to us in understanding the world, we make what is, ironically, a glaring error of logic. We forget that performing arithmetic is hardly any more the purpose of a human mind than making a wake is the purpose of an ocean liner. The purpose of the human mind, which the evolutionary forces of millions of years have operated to perfect, is to model the world. Brains only compute as a by-product of their modelling; computers only model as a by-product of their computing.

It is important to recognize that there is a fundamental inequality in the comparison here. Ability in computing can be measured and compared directly – indeed that is exactly the kind of thing that computers are designed to do – so we *know* how much superior they are to us in this respect. Ability in modelling, on the other hand, can only be judged as an art form, and it is impossible to make absolute comparisons. Nevertheless, when we consider the perfection of other biological systems (you have only to think of the movements of an Olympic gymnast) it seems very likely that the human mind is as nearly perfect in its primary task of modelling the world as any machine could ever be. So, even if we were to succeed in creating such a machine, it would probably be very like a human mind. And we have enough of these already. Or if we haven't we know how to make more.

Maintenance

The automatic maintenance of the ocean of ideas which is our conception of life is the purpose of much that is cleverest in our minds. There are good reasons why these functions are automatic, and therefore unconscious, and therefore forgotten. First, the ideas are too large to fit into the window of consciousness all at once. And second, their maintenance is too important to be left to the vagaries of the will.

Just the same need for maintenance arises with the complex ocean of ideas which defines a society, and exactly the same comments apply. The ocean of infrastructure which underpins society is what really matters, but it is unseen because society focuses its attention exclusively on the beaches of innovation and change.

We are going to hear much more about maintenance in the future. The concentration on the incongruent – the change – and the forgetting of the ocean has reached its apotheosis in the disposable society, the phenomenon of consumerism and the emphasis on surface rather than depth. Greedily we gobble up goodies – our houses, our photograph albums and our rubbish tips full of last year's discarded toys. All the exciting things of life are there on the edges of the ocean, the surf washed up on the beaches.

As we romp along, drunk with the excitement of change, it is gradually becoming more and more difficult for even the cleverest people to ignore the compelling evidence that things are going wrong; that the processes upon which society depends must, in the end, be sustainable; that if we concentrate only on the beaches, the ocean will die; that more and more of the effort of life must in future be directed towards maintaining the artificial systems, technological and organizational, which make our lives possible.

So that is why it is so wrong for people to give up and let others do the job of trying to understand the world for them. Society's collective image of the world is nothing less than a summation of the personal images of countless individuals. If people opt out of the process of forming this image it will be formed by a smaller and smaller and more and more specialized sub-group of individuals. This sub-group will be distinguished principally by its certainty that it is right – and therefore by the probability that it is wrong.

Keep on taking the tablets of stone

While society needs the free minds of individual people, it must also, of course, have rules and conventions, they are largely the things that make a society. We can't all choose the voltage of our electricity supply, or the side of the road we want to drive on. We all have to subjugate our selfish, short-term interests in a host of ways for the long-term interests of each and every one of the hierarchy of groups we belong to; our families, our neighbourhoods, our professional colleagues, all the way up to the world itself. Enlightened self interest (which can be defined as allowing someone to get out of a telephone box so that you can get into it), whether or not it is ultimately the only human motivation, is certainly the only way to live.

Society must have rules, and individuals must have freedom. Defining a rule always excludes a degree of individual freedom and somewhere a balance must be struck. The point is that it is striking the balance, *not* thinking up the rules, which is the difficult bit. In the past the balance was achieved by default, many rules which nobody took seriously – midwives weren't supposed to stitch but actually they often did, old people's wardens were supposed to follow the rules but actually used their common sense etc, etc. Rules, we all knew, were made to be broken.

But now technology is being used to enforce the rules without fail and the detached machinery of law is being used to impose penalties without any understanding of the human reality. Computer systems are *par excellence* machines for the carrying out of rigid rules. As they become more established in our society there is a very grave danger that they will impose standard procedures and rigidity to an unprecedented extent. Many administrative and supervisory functions currently performed by people could and probably will be taken over by automatic audit systems. The important thing is that they should be carefully designed to reflect the real objectives of what is being done or entirely different objectives may be permanently built in. This defining of objectives is a task in which 'ordinary people' must become involved. It is absolutely vital that the narrow perceptions of experts are not cast into tablets of silicone.

None of this is the 'fault' of computers. It was never the sword that killed, but the man who wielded it. I have shown in my practice that computers can encourage independence, individuality and diversity. But there is a great danger that they will be used to impose uniformity and constraints to an undesirable extent. It is up to us to lay down the rules so that computers, and all other aspects of management technology, are developed as liberating tools, not as agents of constricting masters.

Rules for rules
- Rules should always be implemented properly so that they are respected. If a rule has been made to be broken then it has been made badly.
- Rules must never, ever, be made for their own sake or for the sake of change. It is never right, under any circumstances, for rules to be created as a justification for the existence of the rule makers or to satisfy their need for power, authority and status. Rule-makers should be servants of society, not rulers of society; rules should be instruments of informed consensus.
- Rules must always be practical – which means they will often be far less stringent than we think (– and enormously less stringent than a specialist in the particular field would think).
- The number of rules must be kept to an indispensable minimum – which means there will be far fewer than we think (– and enormously fewer than the sum of all the recommendations of all specialists).
- Rules should always be created and applied at the most peripheral level of society possible. The best rules are imposed by the responsible adult on himself and each step away from this ideal must be justified.
- Rules should be *safe minimum baselines* not *impossible ideals*. They should be foundations on which to build, not mountain-tops people exhaust themselves struggling vainly to reach. People are best left choosing their *own* mountains to climb.
- Rules should be designed to set the limits of acceptable behaviour, not to direct the details of behaviour.

The essential point is that rules can never describe life, they can only set the limits.

It is noteworthy that those people who are most thoughtful about the application of rules and most troubled by pointless 'stone checks' are the very ones who are most realistic about their own limitations. Perhaps this is because people who don't think any rules matter aren't worried by foolish ones. A colleague in postgraduate GP education in Wessex, Dr Roger Hillman, showed this with a study of how well doctors' real performance matched up to the rules they thought they applied to themselves. He concluded that, 'The only person who did anything near what he thought he did, was the one who thought he did *least*.'

If this is typical of people in other fields of life, as common sense tells us it is, then it means that rules which are going to be adhered to will have to specify *minimum* standards. These minimum standards, furthermore, will be much lower than the *ideal* standards which central controllers may think desirable. And *very* much lower than those to which some individual enthusiasts will undoubtedly aspire. Otherwise, the very act of imposing the wrong sort of rules will kill the initiative of those people who would previously have sought (sometimes unsuccessfully) to reach far above them.

The balanced way forward

We have seen that there are two possible ways for us to proceed. One is the automated, mechanistic, defined way and the other is the soft, instinctive, natural way. The first can't cope with the complexity of life and provides no reason for living; the second leaves mankind blind, lacking in plan and vulnerable to all sorts of dangers.

So this is where we need human minds to make the balance. Enormous opportunities to improve this balance are opened up by technology. By producing a sort of summation of the thoughts and experiences of the entire world, analogous to the image of the world contained in each of our minds, we have the prospect of a new era of media scale super-understanding and even of media scale super-wisdom. But before we can achieve that we have got to understand media scale super-distortion and grow out of media scale super-selfishness.

Although many people now suspect that civilization is rushing towards the brink of a precipice, they have adopted the short term solution of closing their eyes. 'You worry too much, James, why don't you have a drink?'

Others fix their eyes on one thing, typically the pursuit of their own wealth, and exclude the worrying view ahead. Exclusion, remember, is the enemy, the cop-out from life. The more closed the mind has been, the more traumatic the eventual opening is likely to be, but we have no alternative. We must all open our minds and let in things that are 'not our field'. Individuals in all walks of life have got to use their minds to understand the enormously complex world in which we now live. This is the duty of education in its broadest sense. Part of that educational process takes the form of specialists making the main truths of their disciplines accessible to generalists. I hope that I have made it clear that in my book popularization is a good thing. Many of the most able scientists have shown themselves to be aware of this need, and Stephen Hawking's freshness and clarity in describing advanced contemporary cosmology in the enormously popular 'A Brief History of Time' suggests that *no* subject is too difficult for lay people to at least approach. We need specialists who can contribute simplified models, which are consistent with the main truths of their disciplines, to the common stock of ideas. They must watch so that they can perform the necessary fine-tuning when they see errors in people's understanding of these models. And so must everybody else watch and listen to them.

We need far more mutual respect in the world, with the generalist part of each of us respecting the specialist part of everyone else and vice versa. We must respect the whole system of rational thought which is science and at the same time we must remember its limitations. Mankind is absolutely committed to riding the tiger of science, however great our misgivings at times may be. We are totally dependent on the artificial systems that make our lives possible and if we try to dismount mankind will suffer the usual fate of those who get off tigers.

Human understanding is not a game, it is not just an optional extra in the modern world, a mere luxury which makes life richer, it is absolutely essential for our survival. It is only human understanding and common sense which can combine the hard, rigid world of logic and scientific truth with the soft, vulnerable, inner world of human feelings and passions to make a world which works and in which it is worth living. It is time, I believe, to recognize the fundamental imbalance in this equation, to recognize the fact that we are not comparing like with like when we weigh up facts against feelings, and to realize that if we don't give feelings back their due, and soon, the madness of society is going to get very much worse just as we think we are finally getting everything perfect.

If people can be killed by kindness then certainly society can be killed by progress. If you must sometimes be cruel to be kind, we must sometimes go backwards a little in order to go forwards. The backwards I have in mind is towards a respect for human values and for the common sense and integrity of individual people. Backwards to the personal, local scale where people feel they count and that what they do or don't do is likely to make a difference. We need a simpler society, with fewer rules, not more. With a bias towards individual freedom and diversity and away from restriction and uniformity. Most of all we need to keep technology in its proper place, as the servant of the individual person, not the master. To make use of its enormous potential to enhance life; whilst protecting ourselves from its enormous potential to diminish and imprison us.

13

Epilogue

Three recent examples of the application of the ideas in this book to confrontations with centralized regulation.

'You're not a General Practitioner, you're a general philosopher.'
'Ah, but I haven't got any letters after my name as a philosopher.'
'That doesn't matter, it comes with the wrinkles.'
Conversation with a patient.

The video

I have never been able to bring myself to record a real consultation with a real patient on video. I don't really know why not but it just doesn't seem right to me. It would be like having a video running during an intimate conversation at home with your wife, or when you've gone to a trusted friend for advice. It just seems wrong.

Many GPs disagree with me and video is widely used as a tool in GP education. Trainee GPs on courses of the kind I used to run are often asked to bring in videos of their consultations and all sorts of techniques have been developed for assessing them to help them improve their communication skills.

On our course I always made a point of insisting that this kind of thing was voluntary and (being one myself) I respected the position of the conscientious objectors. The videoing of simulated consultations with actors playing the patients was another matter and I found this useful and completely unobjectionable. I actually scored rather well on this myself, so I could see that it was a valuable technique.

So, the years went by without me actually letting the cameras roll on a real patient in a real surgery. Nobody seemed to mind, and my communication skills, in spite of being thus un-honed, were generally held to be more than adequate for the job in hand. Then came confrontation.

It was after I had resigned as a course organizer in despair at the changes imposed on the National Health Service by Margaret Thatcher's government, but while I was still an accredited trainer. One of the requirements for continued accreditation was an occasional attendance at a residential course at Urchfont, a comfortable retreat in the Wiltshire countryside, which I had enormously enjoyed when I went there on first becoming a trainer.

The problem now was that the course I was being asked to go on required me to bring a video of some of my consultations. I got on the telephone—

> 'Please tell Bob that I don't video my consultations. Does it matter?'
>
> 'Oh yes, quite a few people object, but we do require it. Bob says that they all come round in the end.'
>
> 'Oh does he! Well he's just found someone who won't.'

I withdrew my application and didn't go to the course. And from that instant onward the statement, 'they all come round in the end', became untrue and could never again be truthfully made. A small point you may think, but not insignificant. Who says individuals can't change the world? We can all be Popper's one black swan that disproves, absolutely, the statement, 'All swans are white.'

I would certainly never go as far as to say that a GP who is prepared to video his consultations isn't fit to be a trainer, but I was in this very simple way able to take a stand against it becoming compulsory! I am sure we need *some* trainers who have this view of their relationship with their patients.

When I am told what to stop doing . . .

The changes to the NHS introduced on April Fool's Day 1990 included unprecedented centralized controls on the priorities of GPs in their daily work, just as the sections of this book written prior to that date predicted.

They included requirements to visit all patients over seventy-five years of age at home once every year and carry out a list of specific checks, and also to carry out a routine medical check on all adults once every three years. Careful readers will realize immediately that I was doing both of these things already, at least to some extent. From now on, however, the details were actually enshrined in the law of the land.

I was required, for example, to measure the height of every adult every three years. This, I can tell you, makes a very dull graph. Electrocardiogram (ECG) paper, being long and narrow, has been suggested as a suitable format for a life-time's record, though with the danger that a cursory glance might lead an unwary physician to declare you dead.

As far as the over-seventy-five year checks were concerned, I had almost unique experience having visited and checked all my own over-seventy-five year old patients in order to write my *BMJ* papers about chronic visiting and dependency assessment. I had done it once, as far as I know the only GP to have done so, but the law of the land now required every one of us to do it every year. I knew that the law of the land was requiring the impossible. Just like a contractual obligation to practice without your feet touching the ground – a superficially attractive idea which does not stand up to close examination.

In view of these absurdities, and many more, I wrote to the local employing authority. Popper, again, was the key. 'I will consider doing all these new things when you have told me what I must *stop* doing in order to make time for them. My time and energy are fully occupied. If I do these new things I will have to stop doing other things that I am doing at the moment in order to make time. Thinking up new things to do is easy and fun. Sorting out priorities is the difficult bit and the basis of my professional expertise. When you have told me what to stop doing I will be able to judge whether I would be justified in abdicating my traditional professional role to you.'

The reply came back that they could not tell me what to stop doing and that is how the matter rests four years later. I have continued to decide my own priorities and I have never conceded that any manager has the right to dictate to me.

Just to put the matter on an official footing I recorded the whole correspondence and the outcome in our first annual report (another new requirement – but as I have always held that my practice was open to any inspection I had no particular quarrel with that). I think it is extremely unlikely that anyone has actually read the report, but should there ever be a need to refer to it, there it is in their files, set out just as I have written it here, my justification for continuing to decide my own priorities in caring for my patients.

Unanswerable. Thanks to Popper.

Postgraduate education allowance

Another 1990 April Fool was a new system of Postgraduate Accreditation, reputedly invented by Kenneth Clarke (Minister of Health) himself. GPs get an allowance of about £2000 a year if they attend a certain minimum of postgraduate education – not an unreasonable arrangement you may think.

My first experience of the new system was at the Spring Meeting of the Royal College of General Practitioners in Harrogate in April 1990. The claim sheet which accompanied the programme indicated that of the total of twenty four lectures (in two simultaneous programmes – the 'academic' and the 'scientific') only eighteen had been judged to be of educational value. In each case the regional postgraduate adviser had indicated into which educational category, in his opinion, the subject would fall. So each item on the list had either an 'A' for health promotion/prevention of illness, a 'B' for disease management, or a 'C' for service management. Each lecture counted for one quarter of a day's credit in the assigned category and at the end of the weekend we were to circle the credits we had amassed and send in the form with a cheque for three pounds for each quarter day.

Having grasped the rules of the game, a closer study of the list began to reveal a number of curious anomalies. For example, the Saturday afternoon session in the 'scientific' programme consisted of six papers, only five of which had been approved for quarter-day credits. (The lecture that did not count was the one by a Canadian guest – a foreigner, demmit!) So somebody who sat through that lot got four 'A' credits and a 'B'.

If on the other hand a delegate did what I did and spent the same afternoon in the 'academic' session things were quite different. We heard Sir Roy Griffiths on 'Management in General Practice' – a 'C', Christian Schumaker (yes, the son of the great Fritz) on 'The Good Manager' – another 'C', and Professor James Howie on 'The Measurement of Stress in General Practice' – an 'A'. In other words, we got three quarter-day credits while the others got five. So some delegates had experienced one and a quarter days and the others three quarters of a day, all in the same afternoon. I had thought that this kind of time-dilation effect was only possible during journeys over inter-stellar distances at close to the speed of light. This in itself seemed to me to be a phenomenon of great academic and scientific interest, yet it passed unremarked. Nor did the fact that the two best addresses by far at the conference didn't get any credits at all.

I think it is very demeaning to our profession that anyone should think we only go to academic activities in order to get these ridiculous credits. In fact it is often said that this is the case. But it is now just as untrue as saying that all GPs eventually give in and video their consultations.

I do still take part in educational activities in spite of the fact that I'm not claiming my allowance at all this year. It is worth every penny. I am in the happy position of being able to afford it (partly because better off people pay so scandalously little tax in Britain today) and I now have the luxury of completely by-passing the absurdities of the accreditation process and choosing what I want to do for myself. I am spending this Friday at a day's course on *Microsoft Access*, for example, (which, by avoiding the need for a commercial practice computer system has saved us many times £2000) and I spent my week's study leave last year sitting here at my desk planning my own session for the 1994 RCGP Spring meeting which achieved the first standing applause I have ever seen for a speaker at a medical meeting.

I called the session 'The Paradox of Progress' and subtitled it 'An exploration of the problem of retaining respect for human values in an increasingly systematized world.' Alan Pattison, retired headmaster, put the solution as follows for the benefit of a roomful of spellbound doctors:

'Teaching is very much a matter of having enough freedom, within a reasonable structure, to exercise gifts and judgement. Surely that is what you as GPs must retain: the freedom to exercise personal judgement and to relate to each patient in a personal way.'

That is what this book has been about and I hope it has struck the same chord that we struck in that conference room. Just in time for the millennium.

Booklist

Some books I found helpful . . .

Adams, D (1979) *The Hitch-Hiker's Guide to the Galaxy*. Pan Macmillan, London.
Essential reading for anyone who doesn't yet know 'the answer to the world, the universe and everything'.

Adams, R (1973) *Watership Down*. Puffin, London.
A major inspiration to me in revealing the limits to our perception of large numbers, through the eyes of an appealing colony of rabbits.

Blanchard, K and Johnson, S (1982) *The One Minute Manager*. Berkeley Books, London.
One minute is about the amount of time I have for modern management techniques – but provided you keep them in balance there are lots of good ideas here.

British Medical Association (1987) *Living with Risk The British Medical Association Guide*. John Wiley, London.
A well illustrated guide to putting the relative risks of modern life into rational perspective.

Capra, F (1976) *The Tao of Physics*. Flamingo, London.
The classic account of the extraordinary parallels between contemporary physics and traditional Eastern Mysticism. Typically, I read the sequel, *The Turning Point* (1983) Flamingo, London.

Dawkins, R (1986) *The Blind Watchmaker*. Longman Scientific and Technical Publishing, London.
Another highly accessible book by a prominent scientist. Intended to be a definitive answer to those who question Darwinian evolution it incorporates some of the most beautiful descriptions ever written of the incredible refinement of biological systems.

de Bono, E (1970) *Lateral Thinking*. Penguin, London.
de Bono's ideas only seem obvious when you know them. The richness

and variety of his insights into the generation of new ideas is itself indicative of their efficacy. I always find his books stimulating. Other examples are: *Teaching Thinking* (1978) Pelican; *The Happiness Purpose* (1979) Pelican; *Six Thinking Hats* (1985) Viking and *Water Logic* (1994) Pelican. Pelican publishers and Viking publishers are in London.

Eliot, G (1871) *Middlemarch*. Penguin Classics, London.
I read *Middlemarch* relatively recently but before the television dramatization and was fascinated to find that George Eliot had been thinking about the impact of technology on human values more than a century ago. What is more she knew the answers.

Ellul, J (1964) *The Technological Society*. Vintage, New York. (Originally *La Technique ou l'enjou du siècle*, 1954).
Jacques Ellul was a professor in the Faculty of Law at Bordeaux University and had been a leader of the French Resistance. His book describes what he saw as the tragedy of a civilization in which traditional human values were being usurped relentlessly by the alien forces of technology. He may have been too gloomy and overstated his case, but I'm not sure.

Evans, C (1979) *The Mighty Micro*. Victor Gollancz, London.
I include this out of nostalgia because it was the book which more than any other introduced the British public to the computer revolution, just in time for the Sinclair ZX80; a real computer for £99!

Feynman, R P (1986) *Surely You're Joking, Mr Feynman! Adventures of a Curious Character*. Bantam, London.
Nobel prize-winning theoretical physicist, bongo drummer, painter of nudes, adventurer, teacher, storyteller – a true generalist and one of the great personalities of theoretical physics describes an astonishingly varied selection of incidents from his personal and scientific life with boyish glee.

Gleick, J (1988) *Chaos*. Heinemann, London.
There is much more to chaos theory than pretty patterns and butterflies' wings affecting the weather on Mars; it is fundamental to the emerging understanding of the relations between causes and effects. Good material if you believe that the world can't be modelled in simple formulae.

Gould, S J (1990) *Wonderful Life – The Burgess Shale and the Nature of History*. Hutchinson Radius, London.
A fascinating account of recent fossil discoveries that confounded all expectations and showed that there was a vastly greater diversity of life

forms when animals first began to emerge than there is today, most of the prototypes having been eliminated by natural selection. Gould goes on to a typically far-reaching discussion of how new things develop in general. His books of essays are also excellent.

Gribben, J (1984) *In Search of Schrödinger's Cat.* Corgi, London.
A lucid account of quantum physics by a scientist and professional writer. Purely as an historical account of the emergence of a fantastic new idea it makes for thrilling reading. As an account of how the scientific community now view the world we live in it is more stimulating and astonishing than any fiction.

Hawking, S (1988) *A Brief History of Time.* Bantam, London.
It is sometimes thought smart to say that this is the best seller nobody finishes. Nobody, however, quite manages to shrug off the symbolism of someone who can't speak explaining such profundities so clearly. *Black Holes and Baby Universes and other essays.* (1993) Bantam, London; is also a fascinating read.

Levi, P (1986) *The Periodic Table.* Abacus, London.
A work of superb artistry by a chemist who survived Auschwitz. Levi gives us deft little glimpses of his world in astonishingly contrasted chapters – each taking a different chemical element as its theme. A major inspiration.

Magee, B (1973) *Popper.* Fontana, London.
Not just a concise and clear account of the work of a man whom Sir Peter Medawar, a winner of the Nobel Prize for Medicine, described as, 'incomparably the greatest philosopher of science that has ever been'; but an illustration of how a skilful writer can make knowledge accessible to people who haven't the time or energy to plough through the original texts.

Mill, J S (1859) *On Liberty.* Penguin Classics, London.
'The only purpose for which power can rightfully be exercised over any member of a civilised community, against his will, is to prevent harm to others . . .' The classic account of the importance of individual liberty.

Morrell, D (1965) *The Art of General Practice.* Livingstone, London.
Of the descriptions of general practice I have come across, this is the one I identify most consistently with.

Munthe, A (1975) *The Story of San Michele.* Mayflower. (First published by John Murray (1929) London.)
An extraordinarily poetic autobiography by an outstanding doctor and

man, which enjoyed great popularity earlier this century. The autonomy society allowed to such practitioners in the past obviously stimulated some to greatness, whilst it undeniably allowed others to sink.

Parkinson, C N (1958) *Parkinson's Law or The Pursuit of Happiness.* John Murray, London.
Funny and readable. *Parkinson's law* is now part of our language but we haven't learned a thing.

Penrose, R (1990) *The Emperor's New Mind – concerning computers, minds, and the laws of physics.* Vintage, London.
Roger Penrose's classic argument, using impeccable science, that there are elements of mystery in the workings of the human mind which distinguish it fundamentally from any machine we can conceive of constructing. Reading it I was conscious that I had reached the same conclusion from an entirely different approach.

Pirsig, R M (1974) *Zen and the Art of Motorcycle Maintenance.* Vintage, London.
An indescribable exploration of the interface between art and technology. I also enjoyed *Lila – an inquiry into morals*, Pirsig's eagerly awaited second book which appeared in 1991, published by Bantam Press, London.

Rhodes, P (1976) *The Value of Medicine.* George Allen and Unwin, London.
A scholarly, thoughtful and unusually objective account by a doctor of the purpose of medicine in the modern world. Professor Rhodes was Dean of St Thomas's Hospital and later of the Faculty of Medicine in the University of Adelaide. He was the first to encourage my efforts towards this book when he later became Postgraduate Dean at Southampton Medical School.

Skrabanek, P and McCormick, J (1990) *Follies and Fallacies in Medicine.* Tarragon Press, London.
An inspired, sustained and funny assault on fashionable but unscientific preoccupations in medicine. Rare common sense.

Stoppard, T (1988) *Hapgood.* Faber and Faber, London.
Act 1, scene 2 of this rather baffling play contains a brilliantly lucid account of the uncertainty principle of quantum mechanics – which Richard Feynman described as the *only* mystery. I include this as another example of how we can gain understanding from a blend of art and science.

Toffler, A (1980) *The Third Wave*, Pan Macmillan, London.
Toffler followed *Future Shock* (which I didn't read) with this detailed analysis of where a society goes when it no longer needs most of its members to be working in industry.

Wood, B (1984) *Alias Papa – A Life of Fritz Schumaker.* Oxford Paperbacks, London.
The distinguished economist who left Hitler's Germany before the outbreak of war because, unlike his family and friends (and *Time* magazine), he could not accept what was being done to truth. Originally the epitome of an establishment figure, he was one of the intellectual giants whose authority formed the backbone of the alternative world view as it emerged in the early nineteen seventies.

Having decided to include this list I found I could make it neither short nor complete – two corollaries from what I have said in the text. Thus, although I have included most of the books I have read carefully and found helpful, I am sure I've forgotten others and left out far more into which I only dipped. I have not attempted to include countless magazine and newspaper articles (for example I have subscribed to *New Scientist* weekly for most of my adult life). Nor have I included items gleaned from radio, television or other media. Nor the professional books and journals which are the staple of my trade. I haven't mentioned the many, massive computer manuals that have taught me a succession of languages and programs over the past fourteen years, nor the books about design, gardening, music and all the other things that have contributed to my life as a generalist.